THE SCIENCE OF RED LIGHT THERAPY

YOUR COMPLETE GUIDE FOR HEALING, ANTI-AGING, AND PEAK PERFORMANCE

DR. K.D. CHRISTENSEN

CONTENTS

INTRODUCTION

In the quiet corridors of a bustling hospital, I witnessed a remarkable transformation. A patient who had battled chronic pain for years found relief not through medication, but through the gentle glow of red light therapy. Her journey from agony to comfort was not unique, but it was transformative. Red light therapy has emerged as a promising tool for healing, anti-aging, and enhancing physical performance. This book explores its potential to revolutionize our approach to wellness.

I am Dr. K.D. Christensen, a retired Sports Chiropractor with over 40 years of experience in rehabilitation and holistic health practices. Throughout my career, I have sought effective natural therapies to support my clients' health. Red light therapy stood out as a powerful ally, offering benefits backed by science.

The purpose of this book is to serve as your guide to red light therapy. It is designed to provide a thorough understanding of how to use cutting-edge science to achieve total wellness. Whether you're looking to heal, slow the aging process, or enhance your physical capabilities, this book is for you.

Our audience includes a diverse group of individuals seeking natural health solutions. Seniors, adults, and teens alike will find value in the insights and strategies presented. The broad appeal of red light therapy lies in its ability to address various health concerns across different age groups.

Red light therapy is more than a trend. It is a significant wellness tool with a solid scientific foundation. Research shows that it can stimulate cellular repair, reduce inflammation, and promote overall health. Its applications range from skin rejuvenation to muscle recovery, offering a versatile approach to well-being.

This book delves into key themes such as healing, anti-aging, and performance enhancement. Each chapter explores these themes with a focus on practical applications. You will learn about the mechanisms behind red light therapy and how to integrate it into your wellness routine.

My motivation for writing this book stems from my professional journey and the positive outcomes I've seen in my clients. Over the years, I've watched individuals reclaim their health and vitality through simple, non-invasive therapies. Red light therapy stands out as a particularly effective option, inspiring me to share my knowledge and experiences.

As you journey through this book, prepare to engage with both scientific insights and practical advice. The content is designed to be actionable, providing strategies that you can implement to enhance your health. Whether you're new to red light therapy or looking to deepen your understanding, this book offers valuable guidance.

I encourage you to actively engage with the content. Take notes, experiment with the strategies discussed, and observe the effects on your health. Your proactive approach will maximize the benefits of red light therapy, empowering you to take charge of your wellness journey.

In closing, I invite you to explore the power of red light therapy. Use this book as a tool to enhance your well-being and share your experiences with others. Together, we can harness this remarkable therapy to improve our lives and the lives of those around us. The journey to better health begins here.

1

UNDERSTANDING RED LIGHT THERAPY

In the heart of ancient Egypt, healers harnessed the sun's rays to treat various ailments, steadfast in their belief in the sun's divine power to promote health and vitality. These early practitioners unknowingly pioneered what would eventually become known as light therapy, a method that has evolved significantly over millennia. Today, standing at the threshold of rediscovering these ancient practices, now refined and backed by modern science, we find ourselves equipped with red light therapy—a therapeutic tool with the promise of healing, rejuvenation, and enhanced performance, all firmly grounded in empirical research and technological innovation.

THE HISTORICAL EVOLUTION OF LIGHT THERAPY

The origins of light therapy trace back to a time when ancient civilizations revered the sun not only as a deity but also as a vital source of life-giving energy. The Egyptians, with their profound understanding of natural elements, utilized sunlight in healing rituals, recognizing its potential to invigorate the body and spirit.

This practice laid the groundwork for future explorations into the therapeutic properties of light.

As centuries passed, the appreciation of light continued across cultures. The Greeks and Romans, for example, constructed solariums to harness sunlight's energy for healing purposes, recognizing its benefits long before modern science could explain its workings. During the Renaissance, an era of profound intellectual awakening, there was a renewed interest in the scientific examination of light, setting the stage for its therapeutic applications.

Moving forward to the late 19th century, Danish physician Niels Ryberg Finsen pushed medical science into new realms with his groundbreaking work on light therapy. Finsen's meticulous research on concentrated light radiation led to treatments for diseases such as lupus vulgaris, a debilitating skin condition caused by tuberculosis bacteria. His pioneering efforts were recognized with a Nobel Prize in 1903, marking a pivotal moment in the history of phototherapy. Finsen's contributions validated the therapeutic potential of light and spurred further scientific inquiry into its wide-ranging applications.

Subsequent decades saw significant advancements in phototherapy as medical science embraced new technologies. The mid-20th century marked a quantum leap in therapeutic modalities with the development of lasers and light-emitting diodes (LEDs). Researchers discovered that specific wavelengths of light could target cellular processes with remarkable precision, opening new avenues for medical treatment. This breakthrough paved the way for red light therapy, which employs low-level wavelengths to stimulate cellular repair and regeneration.

The multitude of uses soon became apparent; not only were these therapies addressing dermatological concerns, but they also ventured into fields such as laser eye surgery, cancer treatment, and vitiligo management. The therapeutic application of light was revolutionized with the development of LEDs, allowing for safer, more controlled treatments compared to earlier methods that relied on sunlight or intense artificial sources.

Red light therapy gradually transitioned from an alternative medicine practice to mainstream acceptance. Dermatologists incorporated it into treatments for various skin conditions, leveraging its capacity to accelerate wound healing and enhance collagen production (Healthline). Physical therapists recognized its efficacy in reducing inflammation and promoting recovery in musculoskeletal injuries. As scientific evidence accumulated, red light therapy gained credibility within both medical and wellness communities.

This evolution mirrors a broader trend toward non-invasive therapies that prioritize holistic well-being. In today's wellness landscape, red light therapy stands alongside other complementary approaches such as acupuncture and massage therapy. Its appeal lies in its ability to offer tangible benefits without the risks associated with more invasive procedures. By stimulating natural healing processes at the cellular level, red light therapy empowers individuals to take control of their health.

Recognizing the therapeutic potential of light, various wellness centers and gyms have incorporated this therapy into their offerings. Wellness enthusiasts now use devices at home, customizing their use to suit personal health goals. This democratization of therapy reflects the broader shift towards personalized health and self-care regimens, aligning with other advancements like telemedicine and mobile health apps.

To fully appreciate red light therapy's place within modern wellness practices, consider its versatility and adaptability. Unlike some therapies that require specialized environments or equipment, red light therapy can be easily integrated into your daily routine. Its applications range from skincare to athletic recovery, making it an accessible option for anyone seeking improved vitality and resilience.

This accessibility has made red light therapy a popular topic among beauty bloggers and health influencers, further normalizing its usage and broadening its reach. Various kits are now available, ranging from handheld to full-body set-ups, each tailored to different user needs.

As you explore the intricacies of red light therapy, you'll discover its capacity to transform your health journey. By understanding its historical roots and scientific underpinnings, you gain insight into a powerful tool that bridges ancient wisdom with contemporary innovation. This knowledge equips you to make informed decisions about incorporating red light therapy into your self-care regimen.

This chapter has illuminated the rich history and profound impact of light therapy—a testament to humanity's enduring quest for healing and renewal. From the sun-drenched sands of ancient Egypt to cutting-edge laboratories around the world, light therapy has evolved into a sophisticated science with wide-ranging applications. As you delve deeper into this fascinating field, consider how red light therapy might enrich your own path toward optimal health and well-being.

The narrative continues with an exploration of red light therapy's scientific mechanisms and practical applications. In subsequent chapters, you'll delve into the cellular processes that underpin this remarkable modality and learn how to tailor it to your unique needs. This knowledge empowers you to harness red light therapy's full potential, unlocking new levels of vitality and resilience.

THE SCIENCE BEHIND RED LIGHT: WAVELENGTHS AND EFFECTS

Light, in its myriad forms, dances across the spectrum, presenting both visible and invisible wavelengths. To comprehend red light therapy, we begin with this spectrum. Visible light constitutes the colors we see, while infrared radiation lies just beyond our visual perception. Red light therapy operates in this junction, utilizing wavelengths between 630 to 880 nanometers (nm). This range penetrates skin layers, reaching the cellular level without generating heat. Unlike ultraviolet rays, which can damage skin, these wavelengths stimulate healing processes safely.

Various studies underscore the potency of these wavelengths. Research indicates that red light at specific frequencies affects not only the superficial tissues but also significantly impacts the mitochondria within cells, promoting regeneration and enhancing cellular functions.

The impact of red light on cells is profound. At the heart of every cell lies the mitochondrion, often termed the powerhouse. Red light plays a crucial role here by boosting adenosine triphosphate (ATP) production. ATP serves as the cell's energy currency, vital for repair and regeneration. This stimulation propels cellular activities, enhancing growth and rejuvenation. Moreover, red light reduces oxidative stress by neutralizing free radicals—unstable molecules that can cause cellular damage. This protective effect promotes healthier cells and tissues.

Consider the role of antioxidants in this process, which provide additional protection against oxidative damage. The synergy between red light therapy and an antioxidant-rich diet can optimize results, emphasizing a comprehensive approach to wellness.

Photochemical reactions underpin the interaction between red light and biological tissues. When light photons are absorbed by chromophores within cells, they trigger reactions. Chromophores are molecules that capture light energy. In response, a cascade of biological events unfolds, leading to increased metabolism and protein synthesis. This reaction accelerates the repair of damaged tissues and supports overall cellular function. The intricate dance of photons and chromophores illustrates how red light therapy initiates healing at the molecular level.

This therapy's effects extend beyond individual cells, influencing entire bodily systems. Enhanced circulation is one such systemic effect. By improving blood flow, red light ensures vital nutrients and oxygen reach damaged tissues more efficiently. Increased circulation also facilitates the removal of waste products from cells, aiding detoxification and recovery. Additionally, red light therapy has been shown to reduce inflammation, a common factor in many chronic conditions. By modulating inflammatory responses, it eases pain and accelerates healing.

Consider an individual managing arthritis. With red light therapy, chronic inflammation is reduced, improved circulation minimizes joint stiffness, thereby enhancing mobility and quality of life.

To illustrate these concepts, consider an athlete recovering from a muscle injury. Utilizing red light therapy as part of their rehabilitation regimen can shorten downtime and hasten recovery. With improved circulation and reduced inflammation, the injured area receives adequate resources for repair and recovery. This not only aids physical recuperation but also boosts the athlete's confidence in returning to their sport.

PRACTICAL APPLICATION: CONDUCTING A SELF-ASSESSMENT

Before incorporating red light therapy into your routine, take a moment for introspection. Assess your health goals and current concerns. Are you seeking relief from chronic pain or aiming to rejuvenate your skin? Reflect on your lifestyle and daily habits. Identify areas where red light therapy might complement existing practices. Document your observations in a journal, noting specific outcomes you desire. This reflection clarifies your intentions and helps track progress over time.

Imagine a professional contemplating red light therapy to alleviate stress-induced skin conditions. By maintaining a journal, they notice improvements not only in skin clarity but also in stress levels, indicating broader health benefits.

The science supporting red light therapy is robust, with research continually unveiling new insights into its mechanisms and benefits. Studies indicate that specific wavelengths can influence various cellular processes, making them suitable for targeted treatments (Healthline). As evidence accumulates, it reinforces the legitimacy of red light therapy within the scientific community.

Understanding the wavelengths and effects of red light therapy equips you with the knowledge to make informed decisions about its use. By aligning this understanding with your health objectives, you can unlock its potential to enhance well-being and vitality.

In pursuing optimal health, red light therapy offers a compelling option. Its ability to energize cells and systems underscores its versatility across a spectrum of applications. Whether addressing specific conditions or supporting overall wellness, this science-backed modality empowers you to explore new dimensions of health care.

PHOTOBIOMODULATION (PBM): HOW IT WORKS

Photobiomodulation, or PBM, is a term that encapsulates the intricate dance between light and living cells. It describes a process where photons, the fundamental particles of light, interact with cellular components to trigger beneficial biological responses. Unlike other forms of light therapy, which may involve heat or ionizing radiation, PBM works through non-thermal mechanisms, making it a gentle yet powerful tool for healing. This distinction is crucial because it underscores PBM's safety and specificity in targeting cellular processes. PBM employs specific wavelengths of light, typically in the red or near-infrared spectrum, to penetrate tissues and reach the cellular level without causing harm. By doing so, it activates cellular receptors and initiates a cascade of biological events that promote healing and regeneration.

At the heart of PBM's therapeutic mechanisms lies cellular photoreception. Cells possess photoreceptors, molecules capable of absorbing light and converting it into biochemical signals. This absorption triggers signal transduction pathways, akin to a series of dominoes falling in a precise sequence. These pathways lead to increased production of ATP, the energy currency of cells, enabling them to perform their functions more effectively. PBM also modulates reactive oxygen species, balancing oxidative stress to prevent cellular damage. The result is enhanced cellular metabolism, reduced inflammation, and accelerated tissue repair. It's akin to tuning an orchestra, where each player (or cell) performs optimally, contributing to the overall harmony of the body.

Clinical applications of PBM vividly illustrate its impact across various medical fields. Consider the treatment of chronic wounds, a persistent challenge in healthcare. In a clinical setting, PBM has demonstrated significant efficacy in promoting wound closure and reducing healing time. For instance, patients with diabetic ulcers have benefited from PBM therapy, which enhances collagen synthesis and angiogenesis, leading to faster recovery. Similarly, PBM offers relief for musculoskeletal disorders characterized by pain and inflammation. By targeting pain at its source, PBM reduces discomfort and improves mobility in conditions such as osteoarthritis and chronic back pain. These examples underscore PBM's versatility and effectiveness in diverse therapeutic contexts.

Scientific validation of PBM's effectiveness is robust and growing. Numerous meta-analyses and systematic reviews provide compelling evidence supporting its therapeutic benefits. These studies often highlight PBM's efficacy in reducing pain, accelerating wound healing, and improving functional outcomes in musculoskeletal conditions. For example, a meta-analysis examining PBM's role in pain management revealed consistent positive outcomes across various clinical trials (PMC). These findings are crucial as they provide a solid foundation for understanding PBM's mechanisms and applications. They also offer reassurance to healthcare providers and patients alike about the legitimacy of this therapeutic approach.

Further extending its applications, PBM has shown promise in enhancing cognitive function and mood improvement. Emerging research suggests benefits in managing conditions such as Alzheimer's disease and depression through modulation of brain activity.

In clinical practice, PBM is valued for its non-invasive nature and minimal side effects. It requires no anesthesia or incision, making it an attractive option for patients seeking alternatives to conventional treatments. Moreover, PBM can be tailored to individual needs by adjusting parameters such as wavelength, dosage, and treatment duration. This customization ensures that each patient receives optimal care based on their unique condition and response to therapy.

To further illustrate PBM's potential, consider its application in dermatology. Patients with psoriasis or eczema often experience significant improvements after undergoing PBM sessions. By modulating inflammatory pathways and promoting skin cell regeneration, PBM alleviates symptoms and improves skin texture. This therapeutic effect extends beyond dermatology into sports medicine, where athletes use PBM to enhance performance and recovery. By accelerating muscle repair and reducing fatigue, PBM helps athletes achieve their competitive goals while minimizing injury risk.

The growing body of research supporting PBM continues to expand our understanding of its capabilities. As scientists delve deeper into its mechanisms, new applications emerge across medical specialties. Whether mitigating chronic pain or expediting wound healing, PBM represents a promising frontier in healthcare innovation. Its ability to harness light for therapeutic purposes reflects a profound intersection between science and nature—a convergence that holds immense potential for enhancing human health and well-being.

Through this exploration of photobiomodulation, we uncover a multifaceted tool that transcends traditional therapeutic boundaries. Its capacity to influence cellular behavior underscores its role as a cornerstone of modern medical practice. As we continue to explore and refine its applications, we move closer to unlocking new dimensions of healing and health optimization through the power of light.

DEBUNKING MYTHS: SEPARATING FACT FROM FICTION

In the ever-evolving landscape of wellness and alternative therapies, misconceptions about red light therapy abound. Many of these myths arise from misunderstandings of its scope and limitations. A common fallacy is that red light therapy is a cure-all, capable of resolving any ailment with minimal effort. This oversimplification misleads individuals into expecting outcomes that are not feasible. While red light therapy offers numerous benefits, it is not a panacea. Its effectiveness depends on the condition being treated, the correct application, and individual variability. Recognizing these factors helps set realistic expectations.

Another widespread misconception involves the belief that more exposure equates to better results. This notion can lead to overuse, diminishing the therapy's benefits and potentially causing adverse effects. Like many treatments, red light therapy requires a balanced approach. Finding the right dosage is critical to optimizing its effects while minimizing risks. Understanding this balance ensures users achieve desired outcomes without unintended consequences.

Scientific evidence plays a crucial role in debunking exaggerated claims surrounding red light therapy. Rigorous studies have discredited myths suggesting miraculous transformations without scientific backing. For example, some assert that red light therapy can completely reverse aging, an assertion that lacks empirical support. Controlled trials reveal that while red light therapy can enhance skin health and reduce fine lines, it cannot halt the aging process entirely. Nonetheless, its ability to stimulate collagen production and improve skin elasticity offers genuine benefits for those seeking a more youthful appearance.

The placebo effect often contributes to perceived results in wellness therapies, including red light therapy. This psychological phenomenon occurs when individuals experience improvements simply because they believe a treatment will work. While the placebo effect can enhance treatment outcomes, it underscores the importance of verifying claims through controlled trials. Such studies differentiate genuine therapeutic effects from those influenced by expectation, ensuring the legitimacy of red light therapy's benefits.

In navigating the plethora of information available online, discerning credible sources is paramount. Not all sources offer reliable or accurate insights into red light therapy. Evaluate scientific literature and expert opinions critically, prioritizing peer-reviewed studies and publications. Seek out sources with established expertise in photobiomodulation and related fields. This approach ensures well-informed decisions based on factual evidence rather than anecdotal accounts or marketing hype.

To illustrate, consider a scenario where individuals explore red light therapy for acne treatment. They might encounter testimonials claiming dramatic results after a single session, but scientific research indicates that improvements typically occur over several weeks of consistent use (PMC). By consulting credible studies, individuals can align their expectations with reality, enhancing their satisfaction with the therapy.

Engaging with reputable sources also involves scrutinizing the methodologies used in studies. Reliable research employs randomized controlled trials, which minimize bias and maximize validity. These studies often include control groups receiving placebo treatments to isolate the specific effects of red light therapy. By understanding and valuing such rigorous approaches, users can confidently assess the efficacy of this modality for their needs.

As we dissect these myths and misconceptions, it becomes clear that red light therapy demands a nuanced understanding rooted in scientific inquiry. Its true potential lies in its scientifically validated applications, which offer tangible benefits across various domains of health and well-being. By distinguishing fact from fiction, individuals can unlock the full potential of red light therapy in their pursuit of improved health.

SAFETY FIRST: UNDERSTANDING RISKS AND CONTRAINDICATIONS

When engaging with red light therapy, safety remains paramount. Like any health practice, it demands careful attention to guidelines to maximize benefits while minimizing risks. Recommended exposure times and distances are crucial in this context. Generally, treatment sessions should last between 10 and 20 minutes, depending on the condition being addressed. Maintaining a distance of approximately six to 12 inches from the light source ensures effective penetration without overheating the skin. These parameters are designed to optimize therapeutic effects while safeguarding against potential overexposure. Users should note that increasing either the duration or proximity beyond these recommendations can lead to diminished returns or adverse effects.

The design and quality of red light therapy devices can also influence safety outcomes. Using FDA-approved or medically certified equipment ensures that light emissions meet safety standards, reducing the risk of exposure to harmful levels of radiation.

Red light therapy, though safe for most, is not universally applicable. Individuals with photosensitivity—a heightened sensitivity to light—should approach with caution. Conditions such as lupus or porphyria can exacerbate under light exposure, making red light therapy unsuitable. Similarly, those on medications that increase photosensitivity should consult healthcare providers before beginning treatment. Pregnant women and individuals with severe skin conditions like eczema should also seek professional advice to ensure no contraindications exist. These precautions are not merely bureaucratic hurdles; they are vital for tailoring therapy to individual needs and ensuring safety.

While red light therapy boasts a minimal side effect profile, some users may experience temporary skin redness or irritation. This minor reaction is usually short-lived and resolves quickly without intervention. It reflects the skin's natural response to increased circulation and cellular activity stimulated by the treatment. In rare cases, prolonged exposure might lead to mild discomfort, emphasizing the importance of adhering to recommended guidelines. Users should monitor their reactions, adjusting exposure as needed to maintain comfort and efficacy.

Professional guidance plays an integral role in the successful application of red light therapy. Consulting healthcare providers ensures a personalized approach, taking into account individual health conditions and treatment goals. Doctors and certified therapists possess the expertise to tailor treatment protocols, optimizing outcomes while minimizing risks. Their involvement is particularly crucial for individuals with complex medical histories or those integrating red light therapy into broader health regimens. This collaborative approach fosters a comprehensive understanding of how red light therapy can enhance overall wellness.

Consider a scenario where an individual with chronic joint pain seeks relief through red light therapy. By consulting a healthcare provider, they receive a tailored treatment plan that accounts for their specific condition, medication use, and lifestyle factors. This personalized approach enhances the therapy's effectiveness and provides peace of mind, knowing that the treatment aligns with their unique health profile. Professional oversight ensures that each session contributes positively to their overall well-being.

The importance of professional guidance cannot be overstated. While red light therapy is accessible and user-friendly, its integration into health routines benefits from expert input. Certified therapists provide valuable insights into optimizing treatment parameters, adjusting protocols based on observed responses, and ensuring consistency with broader health objectives. Their role extends beyond mere facilitation; they empower users with knowledge and confidence, fostering an informed approach to wellness.

As users navigate their red light therapy journey, they should remain vigilant about sourcing accurate information from reputable sources. The proliferation of online content can lead to misinformation or exaggerated claims about the therapy's capabilities. Evaluating scientific literature and expert opinions critically ensures well-informed decisions based on factual evidence rather than anecdotal accounts or marketing hype. Users should prioritize peer-reviewed studies and publications with established expertise in photobiomodulation and related fields.

Incorporating red light therapy into one's health regimen involves more than merely acquiring equipment and commencing sessions. It requires a nuanced understanding of safety guidelines, contraindications, and potential side effects—knowledge that empowers users to maximize benefits while minimizing risks. By adhering to recommended practices and seeking professional guidance, individuals can harness the full potential of this innovative therapy safely and effectively.

THE ROLE OF RED LIGHT IN THE BODY'S NATURAL HEALING PROCESSES

Red light therapy plays a pivotal role in supporting the body's inherent healing mechanisms. At its core, this therapy enhances cell proliferation and tissue repair, processes crucial for maintaining health and vitality. When cells are exposed to red light, the energy stimulates growth factors that accelerate cellular replication. This is particularly beneficial for skin rejuvenation, where rapid cell turnover can diminish scars and wrinkles, revealing healthier skin layers. In wound healing, red light catalyzes tissue repair by promoting fibroblast activity—the cells responsible for collagen production. As a result, wounds heal faster, with less scarring. This cellular optimization is akin to a gardener nurturing young plants, ensuring each receives the light and nutrients needed to thrive.

In addition to cosmetic and wound healing applications, red light therapy shows promise in addressing systemic conditions such as autoimmune diseases. Its ability to modulate immune responses and reduce autoimmune flares signifies a potential paradigm shift in the management of such chronic conditions.

Inflammation, a natural defense mechanism, can become problematic when persistent. Red light therapy mitigates this issue by modulating inflammatory cytokines—proteins that signal inflammation. By reducing the levels of pro-inflammatory cytokines while enhancing anti-inflammatory ones, red light therapy restores balance. This modulation alleviates conditions like arthritis, where inflammation leads to chronic pain and stiffness. The therapy acts as a gentle mediator, calming the body's immune response and preventing excessive inflammation. This recalibration enables the body to heal without the burden of prolonged inflammatory stress.

In terms of pain reduction, red light therapy offers a multifaceted approach. It stimulates endorphin release, which are the body's natural painkillers. Increased endorphin levels elevate mood and reduce pain perception, providing relief for chronic pain sufferers. Moreover, red light influences nerve modulation by altering the transmission of pain signals to the brain. This can be particularly effective for neuropathic pain, where traditional painkillers often fall short. By addressing both chemical and neurological pathways, red light therapy offers comprehensive pain management without side effects.

Newer studies are examining its role in improving sleep quality, as reduced pain and heightened relaxation translate into better rest, illustrating its indirect benefits in contributing to circadian rhythm regulation.

The practical benefits of red light therapy are well-documented in various case studies. Athletes frequently turn to red light therapy for its ability to speed up recovery from sports injuries. For instance, after a muscle strain, applying red light reduces downtime by enhancing blood flow and reducing inflammation at the injury site. Similarly, surgical patients have reported faster healing of incisions when incorporating red light therapy into their post-operative care. This accelerates recovery, minimizes infection risk, and improves overall outcomes. These examples underscore the therapy's capacity to expedite healing across diverse scenarios.

To illustrate its impact further, consider a professional athlete who sustains a hamstring injury during training. Incorporating red light therapy into their rehabilitation protocol can significantly reduce recovery time. The targeted application of red light increases circulation and oxygenates the tissue, facilitating faster repair. As a result, the athlete returns to peak performance sooner, with reduced risk of re-injury.

In another scenario, imagine a person recovering from knee surgery using red light therapy to enhance healing. By applying the therapy consistently, they notice reduced swelling and discomfort around the surgical site. Within weeks, mobility improves, allowing them to engage in physical therapy with greater ease. The therapy's ability to enhance tissue repair and reduce inflammation plays a crucial role in their recovery journey.

As the pathway to adoption broadens, many practices now offer integrated light therapy sessions combined with physiotherapy or chiropractic treatments, which further enhances patient outcomes.

Red light therapy's integration into health routines offers a safe and effective means of supporting the body's natural processes. Its potential to optimize cellular function, mitigate inflammation, and alleviate pain positions it as a valuable tool in modern wellness practices. By understanding these mechanisms, individuals can make informed decisions about incorporating red light therapy into their self-care regimens.

The aforementioned insights into red light therapy highlight its transformative role in enhancing the body's natural healing capabilities. With evidence-backed benefits spanning cellular optimization and inflammation reduction to pain management and accelerated recovery, this therapy stands as a testament to the power of light in promoting health and well-being.

As we conclude this exploration of red light therapy's role in natural healing processes, consider how these insights might inform your approach to health. Embrace the knowledge gained here, applying it thoughtfully to enhance your wellness journey.

2

CHOOSING THE RIGHT EQUIPMENT

NAVIGATING THE MARKET: TYPES OF RED LIGHT DEVICES

Imagine stepping into a vibrant marketplace, where a sea of options stretches before you—a bustling bazaar of innovation, each stall beckoning with promises of healing, rejuvenation, and vitality powered by the radiant glow of red light. As a prospective buyer, you are faced with a crucial choice that could define your wellness journey. The diversity in devices is vast, offering tailored solutions to meet an array of needs, ensuring there's an ideal match for every individual. As you peruse these options, aligning your selections with your personal therapy goals and lifestyle becomes crucial.

Handheld devices stand out for their precision and convenience. These compact tools are a testament to modern engineering, specifically designed to target treatment in localized areas such as facial wrinkles or isolated pain points. Imagine gripping a sleek device that fits comfortably in your hand, allowing you to direct focused therapeutic light exactly where it's needed. The portability of these devices is unparalleled, fitting perfectly into your bag, enabling you to administer quick sessions during breaks in your daily schedule. The trade-off, however, often lies in their power output. Typically lower than larger devices, these require patience and consistent usage to manifest significant results. Yet, their precision is invaluable—whether it's tackling a stubborn blemish or soothing a persistently knotted muscle, these devices serve as vital tools in your wellness arsenal.

On the flip side, **panels** present a more comprehensive option. These larger units are designed for full-body exposure, providing a broad spectrum of therapeutic benefits. Picture yourself standing before one of these panels, feeling the gentle warmth and healing energy enveloping every part of your being. While they demand dedicated space within your home environment, the investment is returned manifold through their potent solutions for systemic health issues and holistic wellness enhancements. More than just physical wellness, there's a profound element of self-care involved in dedicating time to basking in this soothing light—a gentle embrace for both body and soul.

Additionally, for those who prioritize convenience above all else, **wearable devices** offer a uniquely compelling option. These innovative gadgets seamlessly integrate into daily routines, often designed as flexible wraps or aesthetic masks. Visualize slipping on a comfortable strap around your wrist or donning a mask as you unwind, allowing the device to effortlessly work while you continue with your activities. Their hands-free nature greatly enhances their appeal; however, effectiveness can vary based on design specifics and employed technology. The versatility to embrace therapy from virtually anywhere—from sitting at your office desk to lounging on your couch—ensures that this practice becomes a gentle ebb and flow woven into the fabric of your life, rather than simply another task on a to-do list.

Each category of device bears its distinctions, complete with unique advantages and constraints. Handheld devices provide the deftness of precise targeting, but may lack the deeper intensity required for more severe physical ailments. Panels radiate power and offer comprehensive coverage, yet require significant commitment in terms of both space and financial investment. Wearables shine with unparalleled convenience, but might not reach the efficacy levels of stationed counterparts when addressing serious conditions. This equilibrium of strength and limitation is what often guides seasoned users' preferences, who recognize that personal context ultimately influences the ensemble of optimal equipment.

The intended scenarios for usage play a crucial role in narrowing down device selection. For personal, at-home use, handhelds and wearables often suffice due to their flexibility and user-friendly interfaces. They cater perfectly to those with bustling schedules who require therapy without disrupting their existing routines. Conversely, professional settings such as clinics or dedicated wellness centers benefit greatly from panels. The superior power output and thorough coverage facilitate efficient treatment of multiple guests, expediting their transformative journeys. Experienced practitioners find panels to dramatically accelerate client turnover, leading to quicker, more visible progress—an attribute highly prized within professional milieus.

Technological progressions within these devices further influence their overall performance and suitability. Many consumer-grade models involve **LED technology**, recognized for delivering safe, effective treatments characterized by lower energy consumption.

Reputation of LEDs is built upon emitting light uniformly, making them ideal choices for frequent use within home environments. Conversely, **laser technology**, prevalent in professional-grade devices, delivers a more concentrated intensity favorable for deeper penetration, designed to address acute conditions. Understanding these distinctions is fundamental to selecting equipment that is best aligned with your healthcare and wellness goals. Manufacturers continue to expand the boundaries of LED capabilities, covering broader spectrums with improved efficacy—an evolving direction that promises much excitement for the future.

Selecting the appropriate equipment requires not just functional understanding, but also aligning with one's personal needs, lifestyle, and health objectives. Whether gravitating towards the precision of handhelds, the expansive reach of panels, or the fluid integration of wearables, each alternative holds remarkable potential. It's essential when making this choice to carefully consider specific health aspirations, your living conditions, and the daily rhythm of life. This thorough contemplation guarantees that your therapy is as personalized and impactful as possible, impeccably tuned to the rhythm of your individual journey.

Reflection Section: Assessing Your Needs

Before proceeding with a purchase, take a moment to reflect on your specific needs and their synergy with your lifestyle. Determine your aims with red light therapy—is it intensive treatment for certain issues or a holistic enhancement of wellness? Assess factors such as available space within your home and the allocated time necessary for therapy sessions. Matching your selection to these reflections ensures you are better equipped to choose a device that complements your overall goals, seamlessly integrating into your itinerary.

As you navigate this illuminated marketplace, empowered by knowledge and clarity, choosing the right device becomes an exciting, empowering step in enhancing your health and well-being through red light therapy. Consider the therapeutic journeys of friends or family—how their experiences might inform your choice in equipment. Personal journeys can often reveal practical insights that transcend marketing glitz. Word-of-mouth becomes an invaluable guide through this radiant bazaar of options, rich with genuine results.

KEY FEATURES TO CONSIDER: WAVELENGTH, INTENSITY, AND MORE

Unraveling the nuances of red light therapy starts with understanding the significance of wavelengths. Each wavelength performs a unique function, catalyzing distinct reactions within the body. Wavelengths near 630 nanometers, for instance, are optimal for skin rejuvenation, promoting collagen production and minimizing wrinkles. In contrast, wavelengths proximal to 850 nanometers penetrate deeper into tissue, addressing joint discomfort and muscle soreness comprehensively. Recognizing these distinctions is critical when selecting a device aligned with your therapeutic targets. The science hinges on the light's ability to traverse skin layers and stimulate cellular processes that facilitate healing and renewal. Researchers continue to investigate new wavelength bands, with the potential to broaden these therapeutic applications—a promising frontier in this dynamic domain.

ADVANCED CONSIDERATIONS FOR INTENSITY

Intensity significantly influences the success of your red light therapy regimen. Measured in milliwatts per square centimeter (mW/cm^2), intensity dictates the volume of energy penetrating your tissues. Higher intensities can reduce treatment times and amplify efficacy, but they necessitate prudence to circumvent overexposure. Striking a balance between intensity and safety ensures the full spectrum of benefits is realized without negative side effects. Opting for a device with adjustable intensity settings enables personalized treatments, accommodating varying levels of comfort and need. This adjustability proves especially vital for newcomers to the therapy, gradually acclimating them to increased intensities as their skin habituates to the therapeutic light.

DEVICE FORM FACTOR AND APPLICATION

The device's shape and size play pivotal roles in beam coverage, affecting treatment areas and application styles. Smaller devices are ideal for pinpoint treatments, tackling specific areas such as facial spots or localized pains with precision. Conversely, larger devices extend full-body applications, submerging you in therapeutic light for expansive advantages. Consideration of your intended usage guides selection, ensuring it harmonizes with your objectives. The relationship between device size and specific treatment goals dictates whether your focus is on precise, localized results or an overarching wellness approach. Equally noteworthy are the spatial limitations of your living environment; compact apartments might prioritize handhelds or wearables, while larger homes could accommodate more sizable panels.

USER EXPERIENCE AND TECHNOLOGY USABILITY

User interface and ease-of-use substantially augment the therapy dynamic. Devices equipped with intuitive controls and user-friendly settings streamline the process, rendering it accessible regardless of age or technical acumen. From adjusting intensity to selecting session duration, straightforward interfaces minimize potential confusion while maximizing session efficiency. Some advanced models integrate smart technology, permitting control via smartphone apps or voice commands. This integration amplifies convenience, allowing seamless absorption into daily activities, where therapy transitions from chore to ritual.

Evaluating devices necessitates weighing features against personal preference and lifestyle considerations. A device meticulously attuned to your requisites ensures you maximize the benefits of red light therapy sessions. It's not merely about procuring a sophisticated gadget, but rather discovering a functional asset that effortlessly fits your life, enriching wellness and usability. Envision potential shifts in your daily habits upon incorporating such a device—does it become a reflection point, a serene conclusion to your day, or an invigorating ritual greeting sunrise?

Interactive Element: Device Feature Checklist

Craft a checklist detailing your desired features aligned with your aspirations. Include wavelength preferences, intensity levels, and interface functionalities. Utilize this checklist when perusing devices online or in-store, ensuring your choice meets all criteria. Look to incorporate feedback from professionals or trustworthy advisors, enriching your decision-making's substance. A methodical approach secures focus as underlying capabilities evolve, maintaining your trajectory of health aspirations.

By considering these facets, you're equipped with the discernment necessary for informed decisions. Red light therapy devices aren't universal; they incorporate varied features engineered for specific therapeutic exigencies. Mastering these variations positions you to select a device that fulfills expectations while augmenting your wellness journey holistically. Whether it's the faceted targeting of a handheld or the encompassing span of a panel, each choice echoes distinct health pursuits.

This intricate apprehension of key attributes empowers your red light therapy selection process. From comprehending wavelength importance to ease-of-use, each facet frames the therapy's full efficacy. Aligning these elements with personal ambitions paves a course for effective and gratifying experiences. Embrace this journey with conviction, assured each increment is a commitment to perpetual growth and health.

BRAND COMPARISONS: WHICH DEVICE IS RIGHT FOR YOU?

In the sprawling terrain of red light therapy devices, choosing the right brand becomes akin to navigating a lively market's hustle and bustle. Each brand extends unique propositions, underpinned by the bedrock of reputation and market tenure. Established names often boast decades of refinement, contoured by consumer feedback loops, nurturing trustworthiness through concerted innovation. Valuing a brand's stature taps into an expansive experience pool, ensuring your investment is bolstered by assured expertise. Legacy brands project reliability and commitment to evolvement, sustaining assurance through the sector's shifting tides.

User reviews and testimonials significantly influence perceptions of device reliability. Real-world narratives provide insight into product functionality beyond marketing declarations. Common praises encompass efficient outcomes and user simplicity, whereas critiques may underscore issues like brief battery longevity or ineffective customer support. Scrutinizing these reviews garners insight into potential expectations per brand. This dialogic exchange not only informs potential consumers but galvanizes manufacturers toward perpetual refinement. The symbiotic dialogue between brand and consumer is pivotal, continuously steering industry innovation.

Differentiation among brands often stems from unique selling propositions. Some companies heavily invest in proprietary configurations, offering features absent among competitors. For instance, a brand might unveil an exclusive LED array to enhance light infusion, augmenting therapeutic deliverables substantially. Another may integrate app-driven smart technologies for customized plans. Such innovations cultivate brand identity, enabling niche carve-outs within the industry. When evaluating brands, contemplate which exclusive features correspond to your preferences and therapeutic requirements.

Concord between brand choice, budgetary considerations, and intended usage is critical. While some brands market themselves as premium providers with prices to match, others posit affordable alternatives without compromising on quality. Evaluating financial thresholds alongside feature desirability ensures acquisition of desired attributes within fiscal bounds. For those seeking convenience predominately, prioritizing intuitive design and compact dimensions may override advanced technological allure. Align immediate needs against broader strategies—occasionally, modest start-up investments yield expansive health returns.

Renowned brands like Joovv and PlatinumLED enjoy prominence for robust construction and user satisfaction assurances. Joovv, for instance, is distinguished for its modular designs, allowing users to expand their setup aligned with evolving ambitions. This adaptability is invaluable as users aim to scale regimens over time. Conversely, PlatinumLED spotlights elevated intensity and effectiveness, appealing to users stretching for potent treatments over streamlined, shorter intervals. Their devices often offer adjustable settings, addressing diverse goals. These brands exemplify excellence in fashioning versatile groundwork that gracefully amplifies user ambition.

Budget-conscious consumers find solace with options like Rouge and Mito Red Light. Rouge prioritizes accessible pricing coupled with effective therapy, bundling devices with educational materials to amplify user benefit. Mito Red Light emphasizes providing high-caliber devices focusing on essentials, guaranteeing reliable performance without extravagant expenditure. These brands epitomize balance, exemplifying affordability need not hinder efficacy or satisfaction. When prioritizing both function and form, these offerings deliver powerfully compact performances, elegantly sidestepping excesses.

In professional environments, brands such as LightStim and Celluma predominantly serve thanks to their clinical-grade standard and extensive supportive services. LightStim garners acclaim for ergonomic models suitable for dermatological through to musculoskeletal applications. Celluma distinguishes itself with FDA-endorsed customizable light settings suitable for defined conditions. Commitment to research-grounded innovation instills confidence among practitioners reliant on robust, reliable devices for patient well-being. Highlighting brand credibility and expertise is fundamental in professional settings, befitting thorough performance expectations under rigor.

As you survey the brand spectrum, reflect upon priorities—whether they reside with avant-garde tech, user accessibility, or cost-efficiency. Consider alignment with lifestyle and health objectives, informed through user feedback, gauging reliability and performance through collective wisdom over marketing spin. Contemplating these factors leaves you well-prepared to select a brand meeting need, enhancing the overall red light therapy ambit.

The undercurrent of red light therapy's expanding market is vibrant and bustling, with newer entrants challenging the incumbents. Yet, established brands hold steadfast advantage through consistent quality and consumer trust. Armed with variance familiarity and personalized priority recognition, you effortlessly navigate the dynamic marketplace toward devices advancing wellness goals with precision. Through meticulous and informed choice, demystifying brand selection becomes less a matter of choice fatigue and more an enthusiastic embrace of wellness journeys in red light therapy's luminous glow.

BUDGET-FRIENDLY OPTIONS: QUALITY WITHOUT BREAKING THE BANK

In an era of diverse offerings, procuring budget-friendly yet quality red light therapy devices is within easier reach than ever before. Many manufacturers adeptly craft devices strikingly between affordability and practical functionality, sculpting reliable solutions that sustain practical results without destructive price tags. Brands such as Rouge and Mito Red Light have carved respectable niches, prioritizing key features supporting efficacious therapy whilst remaining saliently accessible. These brands cleverly streamline aspects pivotal to therapeutic success while curtailing costs—sophistication often achieved through simplicity; a sturdy aide capable of remarkable feats.

When scouting devices, evaluate the features-to-price balance. This involves assessing device capabilities versus cost, discerning comprehensive value. Devices like Solawave's 4-in-1 Radiant Renewal Skincare Wand exemplify efficiency through versatile performances at reasonable cost points. Combining red light therapy with microcurrent stimulation, among other functionalities, it delivers robust skincare solutions without multiple hardware investments. Its compact design and seamless ease of use characterize it as an ideal candidate for those entailing efficiency and efficacy within their wellness pursuits. Here, amalgamating features keeps cost-effective rationale at the forefront—a hallmark of utility through clarity.

To further enrich accessibility of red light therapy, many enterprises extend flexible financing and discount opportunities. Financing arrangements diffuse cost across several months, alleviating financial impetuses linked to higher-quality equipment. Collaborative ventures with financing facilitators offer interest-free installment plans, flattening budget bumps while investing in health. Moreover, strategic discount promotions melded with holiday events effectively mitigate costs, allowing access to premium devices considerably beneath standard pricing. Such incentivizing strategies highlight an acute brand intuition to steer clear of restricting consumer access amidst economic variance.

Durability and associated warranties are paramount considerations when navigating budget-friendly selections. Lengthier warranties reflect manufacturer confidence in device longevity and robustness. Numerous budget-conscious models now envelop warranties extending three years, insulating owner investments against manufacturing glitches. Reassurance accompanies such guarantees, aligning device value perception with tangible product resilience. Long-lasting propositions render initial acquisitions far more justified with fewer replacement connotations. Thoughtful consumerism results in a foresight-rich expenditure destined for prolonged relevance over time.

Red light therapy device investments should equally forecast long-term benefits. While initial outlays may appear daunting, contemplate potential return on investment (ROI) in health improvements. Regular device utilization fosters integral enhancements in skin vitality, pain management, and overarching wellness. By lessening dependence on expensive skincare, devices single out medical costs effectively as partnerships in health. This paradigm shifts away from monetary outlays, highlighting cumulative benefits, emphasizing devices' contribution to ongoing wellness commitments, and health stewardship.

Beyond fiscal benefits, potential health improvements are predictive of enriched life quality. Consistency in utilizing red light therapy potentially alleviates varying physiological concerns while enhancing vigor. Individuals grappling with chronic conditions might enjoy reduced discomfort, affording wider participation in daily engagements. Those targeting skincare ambitions can rejuvenate skin naturally sans invasive treatments. The device's health footprint could be as profound as promoting a certain and worthwhile forward-mindedness in health overtures.

Ultimately, recognizing budget-friendly red light therapy demands precise considerations. Focusing on optimal functionalities without compromising essentials optimizes value over ostentation. Financing options and warranty assurances ensure broader access with ongoing peace of mind, rendering strategic, informed choices possible. Recognizing that effective solutions can still lie within financial constraints fosters accessibility to these transformative tools. These devices, adaptable and efficient, demonstrate that innovation in health technology can remain equitable, further enriching life's tapestry with vibrant wellness.

3

APPLICATION PROTOCOLS FOR SKIN HEALTH

REDUCING WRINKLES AND FINE LINES: A STEP-BY-STEP GUIDE

Imagine gazing into the mirror, only to see a rejuvenated reflection staring back at you, with wrinkles and fine lines softened and skin radiating a youthful glow. The magic of this transformation stems from red light therapy, an approach amalgamating age-old wisdom with cutting-edge science. To begin this journey of renewal, establishing a consistent regimen is essential. Aim to set aside 10-15 minutes for a red light therapy session each morning, a time when your skin tends to be most responsive. Engage with the device at a comfortable distance of about six to twelve inches, allowing the gentle illumination to delicately embrace your skin. This proximity ensures effective penetration without discomfort. Repeat this routine three to five times a week, slowly increasing the frequency as your skin becomes accustomed to the treatment.

Complementary skincare habits can greatly amplify the benefits of red light therapy. Following each session, applying a hydrating serum rich in antioxidants is pivotal. Antioxidants counter oxidative stress—one of the primary culprits of aging—while serums enhance the absorption of light-induced energy, nourishing the skin at a cellular level. Capture moisture with a high-caliber moisturizer to keep skin supple and resilient throughout the day. This duo acts as a protective barrier, shielding the skin from environmental aggressors and maximizing the therapy's impact.

Patience is key in witnessing results. Initial skin texture improvements often become evident after two weeks. You might notice a subtle smoothness, as though your skin has awakened from dormancy. Yet, significant transformations take time. Expect to see peak improvements after eight to twelve weeks, aligning with the natural cycle of skin regeneration for optimal outcomes.

Safety concerns often arise with the incorporation of new treatments, more so for aging skin. Red light therapy remains non-invasive, with minimal risk of side effects. However, some users report temporary redness or slight sensitivity post-treatment. To mitigate this, consider applying a cooling mask or soothing gel to calm the skin, reducing inflammation and enhancing comfort.

Reflection Section: Tracking Your Progress

Implementing a skincare journal could be invaluable as you embark on your red light therapy journey. Document details such as session duration, frequency, and any discernible changes in skin texture. Note even the subtle shifts, like increased brightness or elasticity. Over time, these entries offer insights into your progress and can refine your regimen for maximum benefit. A detailed chronicle allows precise adjustments, targeting the most effective aspects of your skincare routine.

Additionally, you might consider using a dedicated app designed to track skincare treatments and progress over time, allowing for a digital archive that can be analyzed for trends and outcomes. This type of record can also be easily shared with a dermatologist if professional insights or adjustments are needed.

As you integrate red light therapy into your daily routine, remember its potential to transform not just your appearance, but also your confidence and overall well-being. Much like an artist perfecting their craft, each session represents a self-care commitment, reinforcing your dedication to maintaining youthful vitality. With patience and consistency, the gentle illumination of red light can light your pathway to more radiant, healthier skin.

BOOSTING COLLAGEN PRODUCTION: ACHIEVING A YOUTHFUL GLOW

Think of your skin as a finely woven tapestry, supported by threads of collagen that confer structure and elasticity. With time, these threads thin, leading to sagging and wrinkles. Collagen, a critical protein, facilitates skin firmness and resilience. Red light therapy incites collagen synthesis, enhancing your skin's appearance by invigorating fibroblasts—cells responsible for collagen production. These fibroblasts labor tirelessly beneath the surface, creating a network supporting your skin's architecture.

To optimize collagen production, adhere to a protocol crafted for your needs. Select a device that emits wavelengths between 630 and 850 nanometers, effective for penetrating the skin and activating fibroblasts. Aim for sessions lasting between 10 and 20 minutes, three to five times weekly. During treatment, position the device six to twelve inches from the target area to ensure effective absorption. Consistency is crucial; regular exposure encourages the gradual build-up of collagen fibers, strengthening your skin's foundation.

Dietary support complements red light therapy by enhancing collagen synthesis from within. Vitamin C plays a pivotal role in collagen production, acting as a cofactor in the enzymatic reactions that stabilize and cross-link collagen molecules. Incorporate vitamin C-rich foods like citrus fruits, strawberries, and bell peppers into your diet. Amino acids such as proline and glycine also prove crucial, serving as collagen's building blocks. These are found in protein-rich foods such as chicken, fish, and egg whites.

Consider further supplementing your diet with collagen peptides, which are readily absorbed and help provide the necessary tools for your body to maintain collagen production. Research indicates that collagen supplements can improve skin elasticity and hydration—key factors in maintaining a youthful glow.

Imagine visualizing the transformation within your skin's structure. Initially, you might see loosely arranged fibers with gaps. As red light therapy stimulates collagen production, these fibers become denser and more intertwined, creating a robust framework supporting skin elasticity. After consistently adhering to your regimen for several weeks, expect significant improvements in skin texture and firmness.

VISUALIZATION IN PROGRESS TRACKING

To get a clearer picture of the changes occurring, consider photographing your skin under the same lighting conditions each week. This visual progress report allows you to see shifts in skin texture and firmness, providing tangible evidence of improvements. Collagen's rejuvenating effects extend beyond sheer aesthetics. As skin texture improves, you're likely to witness enhanced hydration and a reduction in fine lines. Collagen-rich skin reflects light evenly, imparting a natural glow that signifies health and vitality. This glow boosts confidence and exemplifies the synergy between external treatments and internal nourishment.

To further demystify this process, consider exploring diagrams illustrating before-and-after collagen structure representations. These visuals grant a clearer perspective of how red light therapy influences your skin's intricate collagen web. Observing this progression offers insight into the gradual, impactful changes occurring beneath the surface.

In conclusion to this section, embrace the potent synergy of red light therapy coupled with nutritional support to unlock firmer, youthful skin. By comprehending collagen's role and adopting a comprehensive approach to enhance it, you pave the path for lasting transformation. As you integrate these practices into your routine, remember that patience and consistency are your allies on this rejuvenation journey.

TREATING ACNE AND SKIN CONDITIONS: PROTOCOLS FOR CLEAR SKIN

Acne represents a common, albeit often frustrating condition, affecting individuals across all age groups. The relentless battle against acne can be daunting, yet red light therapy offers a promising approach to managing it effectively. Specific protocols enhance the efficacy of targeting acne, especially hormonal and cystic types. Begin by focusing on affected areas with a device capable of emitting wavelengths between 600 and 700 nanometers. This range penetrates the skin effectively, curbing inflammation and bacterial presence central to acne formation. Consistency is vital—target sessions lasting about 15 minutes, repeated three to five times weekly. Position the device six inches from the skin to ensure optimal exposure without discomfort.

Red light therapy's science reveals its cellular-level impact on acne. By reducing sebum production, it addresses one of acne's primary contributors. Sebum, an oily substance from sebaceous glands, can clog pores when overproduced, leading to acne lesions. The therapy regulates sebum output, maintaining skin balance and preventing blockage. Furthermore, its antibacterial properties inhibit the growth of Propionibacterium acnes, the bacteria causing many acne outbreaks. This dual action—controlling sebum and bacteria—significantly lessens acne severity and averts future flare-ups.

To augment these benefits, consider integrating a gentle exfoliant to prevent clogged pores and enhance absorption of red light. Products containing salicylic acid or glycolic acid can be effective, aiding in resurfacing the skin and maintaining clarity. Also, a non-comedogenic, lightweight moisturizer helps strike a balance, maintaining hydration without exacerbating acne.

Real-life examples underscore red light therapy's potential in transforming skin health. Consider Emma, a 22-year-old college student grappling with persistent cystic acne. After integrating red light therapy into her skincare regime, she observed a pronounced reduction in breakout frequency within two months, with her skin appearing clearer and less inflamed. Her confidence soared, highlighting how red light therapy can markedly improve both skin health and self-esteem.

Beyond acne, red light therapy extends benefits to other skin conditions like eczema and psoriasis. For eczema, often characterized by dry, itchy patches, the therapy soothes irritation and promotes healing. Sessions should last around 10 minutes, two to three times weekly, targeting inflamed areas. In psoriasis cases, red light therapy helps regulate skin cell production, mitigating scaly patches and discomfort. Longer sessions of about 15 minutes are recommended, with a frequency of three to four times per week.

Managing these conditions necessitates realistic expectations vis-a-vis timelines. While some users witness initial improvements within weeks, significant changes typically entail several months of consistent use. This commitment mirrors skin regeneration and healing processes' natural pace. For those with sensitive skin or concerns about potential redness post-treatment, applying soothing moisturizers or aloe vera gel may alleviate irritation.

CASE STUDY: EMMA'S EXPERIENCE WITH RED LIGHT THERAPY

Emma's red light therapy journey underscores its transformative potency for acne sufferers. Initially skeptical, she embraced the therapy after friends' recommendations. Within weeks, redness subsided, and cystic breakouts diminished. Buoyed by these improvements, Emma maintained her regimen diligently. Over time, her skin cleared significantly, boosting her confidence and allowing her to engage more freely in social activities, unfettered by visible acne flare-ups.

Her case exemplifies how red light therapy fits into a comprehensive acne management plan. Emma did not rely solely on therapy; she maintained a balanced diet, rich in omega fatty acids and antioxidant-rich foods to support skin health from the inside out. Her daily regimen included morning and evening cleansing, and she regularly adjusted her routine in response to her skin's needs, showcasing how tailored adaptations contribute to her success.

Incorporating red light therapy into your skincare regimen goes beyond merely addressing individual blemishes—it's about espousing an integrative approach to skin health. By understanding this technology's interaction with your skin's biology, you can tailor protocols to maximize benefits and enhance overall well-being. Whether managing acne or alleviating conditions like eczema and psoriasis, red light therapy represents a versatile skincare arsenal tool.

MANAGING HYPERPIGMENTATION: LIGHTENING DARK SPOTS

Hyperpigmentation typically manifests as unwelcome dark spots, stemming from excess melanin production. Common triggers include prolonged sun exposure and hormonal shifts during pregnancy or menopause. UV ray absorption prompts increased melanin production as a skin defense, leading to uneven pigmentation. Hormonal changes may exacerbate this, altering the skin's natural processes. Enter red light therapy—a non-invasive solution tackling stubborn spots. It penetrates the skin with wavelengths stimulating cellular repair and regeneration, evening skin tone and reducing discoloration. This process gradually diminishes hyperpigmentation, promoting more effective cell renewal.

Adhering to a consistent red light therapy regimen is vital for diminishing dark spots. Begin with sessions lasting approximately 10 to 20 minutes, three to five times a week, spaced evenly for optimal results. Position the device around six inches from your face, ensuring effective skin penetration. While initial improvements may emerge within weeks, significant dark spot reduction usually spans several months of consistent treatment. It's akin to cultivating a garden—each session planting seeds of change, slowly blossoming into visible results.

Enhancing red light therapy's efficacy by coupling it with topical treatments is beneficial. Brightening creams and serums containing vitamin C, niacinamide, or licorice extract can amplify effects by targeting melanin production directly. Apply these products post-treatment, ensuring deeper active ingredient absorption when the skin is most receptive. This synergy creates an effect that accelerates results. Additionally, incorporating a broad-spectrum sunscreen is non-negotiable to shield against UV rays, preventing further pigmentation and preserving therapy gains.

Defining success in tackling dark spots involves setting realistic expectations, understanding skin regeneration's gradual nature. Initially, you might notice a general brightening of your complexion as dark spots subtly fade. Over weeks and months, these spots will lighten, blending more seamlessly with your surrounding skin. Complete hyperpigmentation eradication may be elusive, but significant uniformity and clarity improvements are achievable with consistent care. Celebrate small victories—each fading spot represents your dedication and patience.

Integrating lifestyle changes, such as wearing protective clothing and seeking shade during peak sunlight hours, reinforces red light therapy results. These practices aid in reducing further hyperpigmentation triggers, ensuring that the improvements achieved are enduring.

In your clearer skin quest, common safety and efficacy concerns with red light therapy for hyperpigmentation might arise. Rest assured, this modality is broadly safe across skin types, with minimal adverse effect risks. Some might feel mild warmth or tingling during sessions, typically temporary and benign. Always perform a patch test before commencing treatment to ensure skin compatibility. If discomfort persists, reduce session duration or frequency until your skin acclimates.

Monitor your progress closely, photographing your skin regularly to track changes. This visual documentation serves as motivation and a valuable tool for adjusting your routine. Should you experience progress plateaus, consult a dermatologist for personalized guidance. Their expertise can offer insights into additional treatments or regimen adjustments, enhancing results.

By employing these strategies in your skincare regimen, you arm yourself against hyperpigmentation. Red light therapy exemplifies modern skincare innovation, offering hope and tangible improvements to those seeking dark spot relief. Embrace consistency, patience, and a holistic approach as you strive for a more even, radiant complexion.

INCORPORATING RED LIGHT INTO YOUR SKINCARE ROUTINE

Integrating red light therapy into your skincare routine can transform, boosting current product and practice efficacy. Start by considering session timing. Ideally, red light therapy should follow cleansing but precede serum and moisturizer application, ensuring skin free from impurities and light penetration efficacy. Post-cleanse, apply red light therapy for 10-15 minutes, priming your skin to better absorb subsequent product active ingredients, maximizing benefits and fostering vibrancy.

The synergy between red light therapy and skincare products lies in mutual effect enhancement. The therapy increases blood flow and promotes cell turnover, creating an environment where active ingredients perform optimally. For example, applying a vitamin C serum or hyaluronic acid post-session can amplify hydrating and brightening properties. These products penetrate deeper, aided by the enhanced permeability post-therapy. This combination not only heightens product efficacy but extends regimen benefits, setting the stage for healthier, resilient skin.

Adjusting your skincare routine to accommodate red light therapy entails tailoring it to your specific skin type and goals. For oily skin, opt for a lightweight, non-comedogenic moisturizer post-therapy to maintain hydration without pore-clogging. Conversely, dry skin types might benefit from richer creams or facial oils, replenishing moisture and enhancing barrier function. Those targeting concerns like acne or pigmentation should incorporate targeted treatments—retinoids or brightening serums—post-therapy for maximum efficacy.

Consider conducting occasional "self-reviews" every six to eight weeks to assess effectiveness and determine if course adjustments are necessary. This review includes gauging whether your current routine aligns with your evolving skin goals and recalibrating techniques as needed.

Consistency is paramount in realizing desired red light therapy outcomes. Regularity fosters progress and visible results. Tracking your progress provides invaluable insights into effective strategies. Consider maintaining a skincare journal or using an app to document sessions, noting changes in texture, tone, and overall appearance. This practice not only refines your routine but highlights consistent care's cumulative impact. By periodically reviewing records, you identify patterns and make informed regimen adjustments.

While incorporating red light therapy into your skincare routine, remain open to evolving approaches. Skin responds uniquely to treatments; what works today might need future adjustments. Pay attention to how your skin feels and reacts post-therapy; this feedback is crucial for routine optimization. Should you notice irritation or discomfort, consider scaling back session frequency or consulting a skincare professional.

Red light therapy lends itself to diverse routine adaptation, catering to individual needs while enhancing skin health. Its seamless product integration offers a rejuvenated skin path that feels as good as it looks. By embracing this synergy and maintaining consistency, you unlock red light therapy and skincare regimen potential, paving a path to radiant, healthy skin reflecting dedication and care.

SUCCESS STORIES: REAL-LIFE TRANSFORMATIONS IN SKIN HEALTH

The transformative power of red light therapy has changed many lives, proving its efficacy in reshaping skin health beyond the surface. Margaret, a vibrant 70-year-old, battled deep facial wrinkles. After consistent red light treatments, her skin, once etched by time, exhibited newfound vitality. Margaret noted wrinkle depth reduction and an even skin tone unseen in years. Her story highlights the therapy's potential to rejuvenate aging skin, restoring appearance and self-confidence.

Contrast that with Jake, a teenager navigating acne's challenges. Initially skeptical, Jake had tried various unsuccessful solutions before discovering red light therapy. Over weeks, the angry redness diminished, and his skin cleared considerably. This transformation was more profound than physical; it restored his confidence to freely engage socially, free from the self-consciousness teenage acne often induces. Jake's experience underscores the therapy's efficacy across age and skin type spectrums, proving it caters to diverse needs.

Assessing these transformations reveals measurable results. Enhancements in wrinkle depth and skin tone uniformity are evident, alongside improved overall skin texture and health. Often quantified through dermatological assessments, many users note significant elasticity and hydration level improvements, offering reassurance to those pursuing similar paths—evidence that technology and perseverance yield promising results.

Beyond physical transformations, the emotional impacts are profound. Improved skin health for individuals like Margaret and Jake correlates with heightened self-esteem and a renewed zest for life. Margaret expressed how her enhanced appearance prompted her to reconnect socially, embracing new opportunities. Similarly, Jake actively participated in school events and sports, no longer hindered by acne-induced insecurity. This confidence boost underscores red light therapy's potential as a cosmetic tool and catalyst for positive lifestyle changes.

Documenting these journeys through before-and-after images provides compelling visual red light therapy transformation evidence. High-quality images capture subtle yet significant improvements, illustrating the therapy's real-time efficacy. These snapshots serve as potent motivators, offering a glimpse into what technology and dedication achieve together.

Additionally, sharing stories within community forums or social media groups can amplify the motivation and provide a support network, encouraging others to embark on their healing journeys. This shared experience fosters a sense of community and spreads awareness about the real benefits of innovative skincare therapies like red light therapy.

Margaret and Jake's stories transcend isolated successes, representing a broader hope narrative for those seeking enhanced skin health. While each journey is unique, shared triumphs emphasize red light therapy's universal appeal. The technology addresses diverse concerns, making it inclusive for those committed to skin condition improvement.

Red light therapy is more than a treatment; it's a well-being quest partner. By embracing the technology and integrating it into routines, individuals unlock newfound confidence and vitality, transforming skin and enriching lives with purpose and engagement.

In closing this chapter on skin health success stories, remember each transformation is part of a larger wellness tapestry. These narratives illustrate technology's life-enhancing potential when aligned with personal dedication. As we explore further red light therapy applications in the next chapter, consider how these insights might inspire your health and vitality path.

4

ENHANCING PHYSICAL PERFORMANCE AND RECOVERY

PRE-WORKOUT BOOST: PREPARING MUSCLES WITH RED LIGHT

Imagine standing at the threshold of a significant challenge: your muscles are as taut as bowstrings, your body is a coiled spring ready to unleash dynamic movement, and you're mentally honed for peak performance. This scenario is familiar to athletes ranging from seasoned professionals to enthusiastic amateurs, all of whom continuously explore avenues to amplify their physical prowess. Among the plethora of methods available, red light therapy emerges prominently as a compelling ally. This approach transcends conventional techniques by not only optimizing performance, but also intricately preparing muscles for the demands of physical exertion.

At the core of red light therapy's transformative power lies its multifaceted physiological benefits. Chiefly, it enhances blood flow, ensuring an amplified delivery of oxygen and essential nutrients to muscle tissue. This optimized circulation ensures that muscles receive ample fuel, significantly lowering the risk of injuries while augmenting performance levels. Visualize applying red light to crucial muscle groups—the warmth stimulating cellular activity like an awakening orchestra, orchestrating a symphony of enhanced circulation and vitality.

Integrating red light therapy into your pre-workout regimen can be a game-changer for engaging in intense physical activity. By exposing targeted muscle groups to specific wavelengths, you can significantly increase flexibility and readiness, laying the groundwork for a more effective session. The steady application of red light not only primes your body physically but mentally clues you in for the athletic feat at hand, enhancing concentration and fortitude. Boosted muscle elasticity and diminished strain facilitate smoother, more efficient movement, effectively equipping you to tackle physical challenges with resilience and vigor.

To employ red light therapy effectively in your pre-workout routine, embark on a focused yet concise protocol. Designate 5 to 10 minutes of red light exposure on pivotal muscle areas—be it the quadriceps and hamstrings for runners or shoulders and arms for swimmers. Position the device at an optimal distance of six to twelve inches from the skin, mindful of ensuring effective light absorption without discomfort. Consistency is paramount; regular application not only maximizes the therapeutic benefits but essentializes your training regimen. The resultant synergy of increased blood flow and muscular readiness furnishes a robust foundation for reaching and sustaining peak performance levels.

Accounts from athletes who have fused this approach into their routines are illuminating. Many report diminished muscle fatigue and enhanced stamina during workouts. For example, a disciplined runner chronicled how the inclusion of red light therapy before her morning runs revolutionized her experience. The runner experienced diminished leg stiffness and a substantial improvement in speed and endurance. Her testimony is part of a growing body of anecdotal evidence endorsing red light therapy's efficacy in elevating athletic performance to new heights. Similarly, a weightlifter recounted how his sessions extended in longevity and resulted in fewer muscle strains, empowering him to safely push personal boundaries.

Interactive Element: Personalized Pre-Workout Routine

Embark on constructing a tailor-made pre-workout regimen incorporating red light therapy. Pinpoint the muscle groups critical to your chosen activity and devise a detailed, step-by-step plan for each session. Meticulously document your experiences in a journal, noting any changes in performance or recovery. By maintaining such personal records, you'll uncover trends and adapt your regimen accordingly, ensuring that the richest benefits are realized over time.

Athletes across varied sectors have discovered the distinct advantages of red light therapy. A noted swimmer acknowledges increased shoulder flexibility, translating to refined strokes and improved pool performance. Similarly, a cyclist has noted enhanced power output during high-intensity rides, attributing these improvements to the preparatory benefits of red light exposure. These anecdotes demonstrate how this therapy caters to diverse athletic requirements, providing bespoke solutions to amplify performance across a wide range of disciplines.

Incorporating red light therapy into pre-workout routines offers a comprehensive approach to physical fitness. By addressing physiological preparedness and mental focus, athletes are empowered to excel while minimizing injury risk. Whether you're aiming to become a professional athlete or simply desire to elevate your fitness routine, this method offers a convenient, effective approach to optimizing physical performance for anyone keen on reaching their full potential.

POST-WORKOUT RECOVERY: REDUCING INFLAMMATION AND SORENESS

Following an intense workout, your body transitions into a critical recovery phase, shifting the focus from exertion to restoration and repair. During this period, red light therapy proves invaluable, offering a scientific framework that accelerates healing and rejuvenates fatigued muscles. A primary benefit lies in its ability to accelerate the clearance of lactic acid, which accumulates during vigorous exercise and often results in muscle fatigue. By boosting circulation, red light therapy aids in swiftly flushing out these metabolic byproducts, effectively easing discomfort associated with muscle soreness. The soothing warmth and energy of red light penetrate your muscles, alleviating stiffness and fostering relaxation.

To optimize post-workout recovery, consider the strategic integration of red light therapy with specialized protocols. Timing constitutes a crucial element; aim to commence red light therapy within 30 minutes of completing your workout session to harness a window of opportunity where muscles are most receptive to healing interventions. Sessions should span 10 to 20 minutes, with a focus on extensively worked muscle groups. For those engaged in regular physical training, a frequency of three to four sessions weekly is advised to maintain optimal benefits and sustain consistent recovery. This regularity helps stabilize immediate recovery needs while contributing to long-term muscle health and resilience.

Red light therapy's therapeutic effects extend beyond physical comfort by facilitating inflammation control, a critical factor in recovery and injury prevention. The therapy modulates pro-inflammatory cytokines—key inflammation signaling molecules within the body. By regulating these cytokines, red light therapy curtails inflammation at the cellular level, promoting swift healing and reducing the risk of injury recurrence. This biological response is particularly vital for athletes and fitness enthusiasts aspiring to maintain top performance without succumbing to overuse injuries.

Empirical studies reinforce red light therapy's efficacy in reducing delayed onset muscle soreness (DOMS), a common post-exercise condition characterized by muscle pain and stiffness 24 to 72 hours post-exertion. Research highlighted in reputable journals documents that participants receiving red light therapy report significantly lower soreness levels than non-recipients. These findings reinforce the therapy's recovery-enhancing role, providing a robust foundation for its inclusion in athletic regimens. The supporting science underlying these positive results imbues practitioners with confidence in the method's reliability and effectiveness. In light of this research, many trainers now include it as a fundamental component of athletes' recovery toolkits, often complementing other recovery modalities such as stretching, hydration, and nutrition.

As you consider incorporating red light therapy into your recovery strategy, contemplate its potential impact on overall well-being. Reductions in muscle soreness and inflammation not only improve your physical state but can also elevate your mental outlook. Fewer aches translate to greater enthusiasm for future workouts, fostering a virtuous cycle of activity and recovery. This balanced approach aligns with a holistic view of health, whereby both body and mind reap the benefits of innovative therapeutic techniques.

Reflection Section: Tracking Your Recovery Progress

Initiate the documentation of your red light therapy experiences in a dedicated journal. Record each session's timing and duration, alongside any noticeable changes in muscle soreness or recovery speed. Over time, such records glean insights into how effectively the therapy supports your post-workout recovery efforts. Establishing a systematic approach to documenting progress enables you to refine your efforts, ensuring the therapy consistently meets your evolving fitness requirements.

Integrating red light therapy into post-workout routines affords a comprehensive framework for managing physical stress and fostering muscular health. By embracing this technology, you can enhance your training capabilities and performance while safeguarding against setbacks related to injuries. The synthesis of scientific rigor and practical application renders red light therapy an invaluable asset for individuals committed to achieving fitness objectives with efficiency and mindfulness.

Consider the broader implications of this therapy on your fitness journey. Privileging recovery with evidence-based methods lays a solid foundation for sustained progress and resilience in physical endeavors. As you delve into the intricacies of red light therapy, let its potential inspire a renewed commitment to personal health and wellness, unlocking new perspectives on what your body is capable of achieving.

ENHANCING ENDURANCE: OPTIMIZING ENERGY AND STAMINA

Imagine standing poised at the starting line of a marathon: each cell in your body vibrates with latent energy, and your mind is finely tuned to the task ahead. Enhancing endurance transcends mere physical exertion; it involves the optimization of energy metabolism crucial for prolonged athletic performance. Red light therapy significantly contributes to this process by augmenting mitochondrial efficiency and amplifying ATP production. Mitochondria, known as the powerhouses of cells, are pivotal in generating ATP—the essential currency of energy. Exposure to red light stimulates mitochondria to accelerate their activity, producing more ATP with the same number of resources. This elevated energy production level can substantially bolster endurance, enabling sustained peak performance across extended periods.

Athletes intent on optimizing their stamina may find incorporating red light therapy into their training regimens transformative. Custom protocols for endurance endeavors like running and cycling entail specified session durations and frequencies. Runners might incorporate 15-minute sessions concentrating on their leg muscles, ensuring proper preparation for the rigorous demands of distance running. Cyclists, navigating diverse physical challenges, could benefit from longer sessions targeting both leg and core muscles, fostering holistic stamina enhancement. Regular red light therapy exposure refines energy utilization and promotes faster recovery between sessions, thus facilitating the consistent pursuit of training objectives.

The effects of red light therapy on endurance athletes are captured through varied case studies. Marathon runners, for example, report increased time-to-exhaustion following the integration of regular red light sessions into their routines. One runner recounted improved pace sustainability and reduced post-race fatigue—achievements attributable to enhanced cellular respiration sparked by heightened mitochondrial efficiency under red light exposure. Such testimonials underscore the noteworthy benefits of incorporating this therapy into an endurance athlete's comprehensive toolkit.

Balancing red light therapy with peak training periods demands meticulous planning. Athletes should carefully schedule therapy sessions during rest days or lighter training days to avert overburdening the body. This careful strategy ensures therapy benefits are optimized without compromising performance during critical training phases. Creating a harmonious synergy between the rigors of training and the restorative effects of therapy is crucial. Incorporating short therapy sessions post intense workouts can preserve energy levels and alleviate fatigue, sustaining overarching training aims.

For practicality in embedding red light therapy into an athlete's schedule, identify specific weekly times for this routine. Consistency is vital, with regular sessions helping maintain mitochondrial efficiency and energy production. Athletes should also attentively monitor bodily responses, modifying session lengths and frequencies in alignment with individual needs and performance goals. Logging energy levels before and after sessions offers valuable insights into the therapy's impact, guiding future adjustments for optimal benefits.

Incorporating red light therapy into an endurance athlete's overall regimen transcends immediate results, fostering long-term enhancements in performance and recovery. Science-backed advantages provide a compelling rationale for its inclusion in training plans, should stamina and energy optimization be prioritized. As one navigates this innovative approach, consider its congruence with athletic goals and the prospect of enhancing endurance capabilities. Beyond tangible performance gains, this deliberate approach cultivates a mindset geared toward progressive training and demonstrable improvements across athletic pursuits.

INJURY REHABILITATION: ACCELERATING HEALING WITH LIGHT

Injuries—whether minor or significant, stem from sports or everyday life—disrupt the body's equilibrium, necessitating a deliberate approach to recovery. Red light therapy presents a promising rehabilitation pathway, expediting the natural healing processes. Injuries often result in tissue damage, provoking inflammation and impaired function. Red light therapy champions tissue repair by stimulating cellular processes that regenerate and mend. This non-invasive strategy targets mitochondria within cells, enhancing energy production and accelerating healing. Increased ATP production invigorates cellular repair mechanisms, fostering expedited recovery from common physical strains and sprains.

Consider the complexity of healing an ankle sprain as a case in point. Red light therapy promotes collagen synthesis and mitigates inflammation—two essential components of tissue regeneration. For those suffering from tendonitis, where repetitive stress causes irritation and discomfort, red light therapy serves to alleviate pain by modulating inflammatory responses and boosting circulation around affected tendons. This dual-action strategy soothes pain while hastening the rehabilitation process, culminating in restored function and mobility.

Incorporating red light therapy into rehabilitation protocols entails targeted application and strategic oversight. Commence sessions soon after injury onset, targeting the injured areas for 10 to 15 minutes per session, two to three times daily. Such regular exposure ensures maximum therapeutic benefits without overwhelming healing tissues. For sprains, concentrate on ligaments encircling crucial joint areas, whereas tendonitis cases should focus on inflamed tendons. Consistency and precision in application foster optimal recovery, reducing downtime and enhancing the rehabilitation outcome significantly.

The use of red light therapy is gaining traction in clinical settings, especially among physiotherapists and sports medicine professionals. This technology supplements traditional rehabilitation methods, creating a holistic treatment plan. In the sports medicine context, athletes benefit from significantly reduced recovery times and markedly improved healing rates. Incorporating red light therapy within protocols offers a comprehensive approach to injury rehabilitation, addressing both symptoms and underlying causes.

Contemplate the compelling story of a professional soccer player encountering a severe knee injury mid-season. The anticipated recovery timeline with conventional treatment alone was daunting, threatening his return to the field. However, integrating red light therapy into his rehabilitation regime expedited progressive recovery. Regular daily sessions targeting his knee facilitated tissue repair and minimized inflammation. Within weeks, he observed significant pain reduction and mobility improvement, allowing resumption of training more swiftly than conventional predictions had forecasted. His accelerated recovery showcases red light therapy's potential in transforming conventional approaches to injury rehabilitation.

These narratives are not isolated; they echo a broader shift towards innovative recovery strategies. Athletes across different levels report similar success stories, illustrating red light therapy's pivotal role in shortening recovery timelines and restoring performance levels sooner than expected. These tailored testimonies highlight the therapy's efficacy within modern rehabilitation practices, offering insights into its revolutionary impact on how injuries are treated.

Rehabilitation isn't solely about physical healing; it's equally about rebuilding confidence and resilience. Knowing that your body is recuperating efficiently offers significant psychological relief. Athletes often face mental barriers during recovery, wary of potential setbacks or performance declines. By accelerating healing through red light therapy, individuals regain physical capability and foster mental fortitude. This holistic recovery approach nurtures a confident return to activity and minimizes re-injury risk.

Incorporating red light therapy into rehabilitation journeys empowers individuals to actively participate in their recovery. It offers a scientifically validated method complementing conventional treatments, delivering an integrated approach to healing. Whether you're an elite athlete or recovering from a routine sprain, red light therapy provides an accessible avenue for accelerated healing, substantially enhancing overall well-being. This advanced tool can mean the difference between an uncertain, prolonged recovery and a deliberate, assured return to comprehensive health and performance levels.

PROTOCOLS FOR SPECIFIC SPORTS: TAILORED APPLICATIONS

Tailoring red light therapy to the distinctive demands inherent in various sports can significantly bolster athletic performance and recovery rates. Each sport presents unique challenges, and adapting red light therapy to meet these specific needs can confer distinct competitive advantages. For football players, dealing with the sport's physicality often results in muscle fatigue and minor injury occurrences. Regular red light therapy sessions focused on large muscle groups—such as quadriceps and calves, conducted multiple times weekly—can aid in maintaining peak physical condition and facilitate effective post-game recovery.

Basketball players, frequently experiencing joint stress and muscle strain due to the sport's dynamic movements, can benefit greatly from targeted sessions on knees and ankles to enhance flexibility and mitigate injury risks. Tennis players, constantly in motion with rapid directional changes, may leverage red light therapy to boost agility by focusing on the lower back and leg muscles. The therapy's prowess in enhancing circulation and reducing muscle tension significantly improves quickness and responsiveness on the court. Likewise, rugby athletes find red light therapy indispensable in managing the sport's physical demands, especially from frequent collisions. Incorporating sessions targeting shoulders, back, and thighs accelerates recovery and fosters effective training.

Professional athletes increasingly recognize red light therapy's value within their training regimens, guided by coaches and trainers who customize its use according to specific sporting requirements. For instance, a prominent football coach has revealed how his team systematically integrates red light therapy into their weekly routine, particularly post-match. Players report decreased fatigue and increased readiness for upcoming training sessions. In basketball, an esteemed trainer has detailed the use of red light therapy to manage chronic knee pain, subsequently enabling athletes to sustain high-performance levels consistently throughout their season. These insights underscore the practical application of red light therapy across diverse sports, highlighting its versatility and efficacy.

Implementing sport-specific red light therapy protocols requires careful synchronization with training and competition schedules. Athletes should strategically plan therapy sessions to complement peak training phases and ensure that therapy support aligns with performance goals without interrupting regular practice or competition routines. For example, football players might position therapy post-game to aid recovery prior to the subsequent training session, while tennis players may integrate brief pre-match sessions to enhance agility and mental focus. Harmonizing these therapy sessions within existing routines ensures benefits are maximized with minimal disruption.

Success in embedding sport-specific red light therapy hinges on thoroughly understanding each sport's demands and addressing them by targeting relevant physiological needs. For contact sports like football or rugby, the focus might be centered on recovery and injury prevention, whereas enhancing flexibility and alleviating muscular tension are pivotal in agility-centric sports like tennis or basketball. Adjusting session durations and frequencies per these objectives ensure comprehensive receipt of red light therapy's benefits, optimizing performance both on and off the field.

Athletes themselves have shared compelling accounts of how they personalize red light therapy according to their specific needs. A seasoned basketball player describes how routine knee-targeting sessions have significantly extended his career by effectively managing recurring pain. Conversely, a dedicated tennis player acknowledges on-court performance improvements following brief agility-targeted sessions integrated within her training cycle. These illustrative real-world examples underscore how personalized red light therapy applications can profoundly influence athletic career longevity and potential.

ATHLETES' EXPERIENCES: PERSONAL STORIES OF SUCCESS

Within the domain of sports, red light therapy's influence has been a pivotal change-agent for countless athletes. From novice enthusiasts to elite professionals, these narratives collectively reflect stories of triumph and transformative success. Consider Sarah, a passionate amateur runner who aspired to improve her marathon timings despite rigorous practicing schedules. Upon assimilating red light therapy into her preparation routine, she noticed a marked increase in both speed and endurance. Sarah found her pace improved substantially, while recovery times shortened sufficiently to enable more effective training. This newfound advantage reinvigorated her passion for running, culminating in personal bests she once deemed beyond reach.

In professional circles, James, a reputable swimmer whose career trajectory had reached a plateau, introduced red light therapy into his training and observed significant gains in strength and speed. The enhanced stroke power resulted in faster completion times in the pool. These advancements sharpened his competitive edge and reignited his will to contest at higher levels. Such physical enhancements had profound psychological effects, boosting his motivation and reinforcing his belief in his potential. This mental renewal proved crucial for his return to peak performance, exemplifying the synergy between physical prowess and psychological resilience.

The psychological impact of elevated physical performance extends beyond competition settings. Athletes like Rachel, an emerging tennis star, recognize that increased strength and agility on the court similarly heighten self-assurance beyond the sporting arena. With game improvement came broader confidence transferable to other life aspects. The perseverance and resilience honed through red light therapy transcended into academic endeavors, demonstrating holistic advantages. For Rachel and others, the physical performance strides achieved through therapy translated into deeply rooted resolve and diligence.

Documenting these transformative journeys offers valuable insights into athletes' efficacious integration of red light therapy. Sarah's systematic approach involved consistent pre- and post-run sessions targeting pertinent muscle groups, while James focused on custom protocols tailored to address specific swimming demands. Rachel's regimen incorporated regular agility and recovery-centric sessions designed to maintain peak abilities—crucial given her demanding schedule. Each athlete's story underscores the merits of personalized strategies that align with focused goals and unique contexts.

These narratives are more than mere anecdotes; they are testimonials showcasing the substantive benefits red light therapy affords. Documented performance improvements—in endurance, strength, or speed—bolstered by data and personal anecdotes affirm its effectiveness. Athletes across different domains attest to the positive impacts experienced through red light therapy, offering compelling evidence of its promising potential. A recurring element within these stories is the openness to explore innovative methods that amplify both physical and mental capabilities.

Embracing novel approaches unlocks doors to sustained excellence and holistic personal development within athletic arenas.

As you reflect on these experiences, acknowledge the wider implications of red light therapy within the sporting context. Its reach extends past physical capabilities, nurturing mental endurance and emotional resilience. Athletes' journeys epitomize the innovation that elevates performance simultaneously fostering personal growth. Their successes act as inspiration for those seeking performance enhancements through innovative, cutting-edge methodologies.

As we close this discourse on enhancing physical performance and recovery, cherish the transformative potential of red light therapy beyond the athletics stage. The narratives showcase its capacity to redefine athletic achievement and personal development in unison. By approaching this technology with curiosity and commitment, you unlock the possibility of unprecedented success and satisfaction. The goal is not solely superior athletic performance but fostering a vibrant, health-focused self that thrives within and beyond the competitive sphere.

This exploration sets the groundwork for further discussions on how red light therapy's applications reach beyond athletic performance into broader health and wellness domains. The possibilities remain expansive, promising benefits extending beyond the playing fields, and touching all facets of life in an inclusive journey toward enhanced well-being.

5

CHRONIC PAIN AND INFLAMMATION MANAGEMENT

UNDERSTANDING PAIN TYPES: TAILORING RED LIGHT APPROACHES

Imagine waking up each day burdened by unrelenting pain. For many, this is a reality that affects daily life and activities. The unpredictability of chronic pain can impose considerable mental and physical strain on individuals. While red light therapy offers relief, its success hinges on understanding your specific type of pain. Pain manifests in myriad forms, each demanding a unique approach. Acute pain, with its sharp, immediate onset, typically signals an injury or sudden trauma. It serves as the body's distress call, alerting you to potential harm. Red light therapy's soothing embrace can aid in reducing inflammation and promoting healing, making it an excellent complement to traditional treatments for acute pain.

In contrast, chronic pain lingers, often without a clear cause, persisting for months or even years. This type of pain does not simply signal damage but becomes an enduring problem itself.

Addressing chronic pain with red light therapy requires patience and a tailored strategy. Its persistent nature means that therapy sessions must be consistent and targeted, focusing on areas of discomfort to gradually restore balance and relief.

Different pain types demand specific approaches to optimize red light therapy's benefits. Neuropathic pain, often described as burning or tingling, arises from nerve damage or dysfunction. Tailoring the wavelength and intensity of red light can significantly improve comfort levels for sufferers. It requires careful modulation of wavelengths to soothe the affected nerves without exacerbating symptoms. Inflammatory pain, common in conditions like rheumatoid arthritis, benefits from red light's unique ability to reduce cytokine levels and inflammation markers, offering a gentle reprieve from swelling and stiffness.

Each type of pain dictates a need for a particular wavelength and intensity to maximize therapeutic efficacy. Shorter wavelengths around 630 nanometers are effective for surface-level issues like skin inflammation or minor injuries. In contrast, deeper penetration is achieved with wavelengths closer to 850 nanometers, suitable for reaching muscles and joints afflicted by chronic pain. Intensity should be adjusted based on the pain's nature and severity, with higher intensities reserved for deeper or more persistent discomforts.

To provide further insight into this nuanced approach, I spoke with Dr. Emily Torres, a renowned pain management specialist with decades of experience in both traditional and alternative therapies. She emphasized the importance of individualizing treatment plans when utilizing red light therapy. According to Dr. Torres, "Understanding the root cause of pain allows us to tailor therapy protocols effectively, ensuring that we address not just the symptoms but the underlying issues as well."

Dr. Torres shared that in her practice, she often sees patients who have struggled with traditional pain management methods. By incorporating red light therapy, she has witnessed significant improvements in their quality of life. One patient, a retiree suffering from chronic neuropathic pain in his legs due to diabetes, experienced profound relief after consistent use of red light therapy tailored specifically to his condition. His story exemplifies how this therapy can bridge the gap where conventional treatments fall short. This personalized approach is critical in managing chronic pain, emphasizing the vital role of customization in therapy.

Interactive Element: Pain Journal Prompt

Consider maintaining a pain journal to track your symptoms before and after red light therapy sessions. Documenting changes in pain levels, frequency, and intensity can help refine your approach over time. This practice not only aids in customizing your therapy but also provides valuable insights into how your body responds to treatment.

A pain journal could include sections for tracking mood, dietary influences, and physical activity levels, all of which can impact pain and therapy outcomes. Over time, patterns may emerge, highlighting specific lifestyle changes that further alleviate discomfort. For instance, noting that pain decreases markedly after an anti-inflammatory dinner or a gentle walk can reinforce positive habits that complement the therapeutic sessions. This level of detail helps in identifying triggers and effective strategies beyond basic therapy.

The journey through chronic pain management can be arduous, but with the right tools and understanding, relief is within reach. Red light therapy offers a beacon of hope for those navigating the complexities of persistent pain. By tailoring approaches based on pain types and leveraging expert insights like those from Dr. Torres, you equip yourself with a powerful ally in your pursuit of wellness and comfort.

In this chapter, we delve into the intricacies of red light therapy as a tool for managing various forms of chronic pain. By understanding the distinctions between acute and chronic pain and identifying specific types like neuropathic and inflammatory pain, you can customize your therapy protocols effectively. Expert insights enrich this exploration, providing you with practical knowledge to enhance your therapeutic journey.

PROTOCOLS FOR ARTHRITIS: EASING JOINT PAIN AND STIFFNESS

Arthritis, a common affliction, often targets the joints, leading to pain and stiffness that can disrupt daily activities. For those wrestling with arthritis, red light therapy presents a beacon of hope. Tailoring therapy protocols for arthritis involves focusing on common areas such as knees, hips, and hands, which are frequently affected. These joints bear the brunt of movement and are prone to inflammation and discomfort. By directing red light to these specific areas, you can effectively target the root of the problem, promoting healing and predicting inflammation.

The mechanisms through which red light therapy alleviates arthritis symptoms are multifaceted. Primarily, it reduces joint inflammation. Inflammation is a natural response to injury or stress, but in arthritis, it becomes chronic, exacerbating pain and stiffness. Red light therapy mitigates this by lowering cytokine levels—proteins that signal inflammation—allowing the body to heal more efficiently. Additionally, it stimulates blood flow to the affected joints, delivering oxygen and nutrients necessary for repair and reducing stiffness. This improved circulation eases pain and enhances joint mobility, providing much-needed relief. The consistent flow of nutrients aids in maintaining the health of cartilage and joint tissues.

To maximize the benefits of red light therapy for arthritis, consider integrating it with complementary strategies. Physical therapy serves as a robust ally in managing arthritis, focusing on strengthening muscles around the joints, thereby reducing strain and improving movement. Combining physical therapy sessions with regular red light therapy can amplify results, offering a holistic approach to symptom management. Another valuable strategy is adopting an anti-inflammatory diet rich in omega-3 fatty acids, antioxidants, and phytonutrients. Foods like salmon, leafy greens, and nuts can help reduce systemic inflammation, potentially enhancing the effects of your therapy sessions. Incorporating Pilates or low-impact exercises can further strengthen the muscular system, supporting the skeletal framework effectively.

The experiences of those who have embraced red light therapy reveal its transformative potential. Consider the story of Susan, a retired teacher who struggled with osteoarthritis in her knees. After incorporating red light therapy into her routine, she noticed a significant reduction in pain and an improvement in her ability to engage in daily activities like gardening and walking her dog. Her testimony underscores the therapy's capacity to restore the quality of life for arthritis sufferers. Similarly, Tom, an avid golfer in his sixties, found relief from debilitating hand stiffness that threatened his passion for the sport. Regular sessions allowed him not only to continue playing but to do so without discomfort.

Further customization of red light therapy for arthritis can include varying session times and incorporating heat application before therapy to enhance absorption. Heat helps in dilating blood vessels, which can improve light penetration and subsequent therapeutic outcomes. This combined approach helps to rapidly reduce stiffness and enhance mobility, providing a more immediate impact on your daily routine.

These personal stories highlight the real-world impact of red light therapy on arthritis management. They provide tangible evidence that this non-invasive treatment can offer significant relief from the burdensome symptoms of arthritis. For many patients, it represents a shift from merely coping with pain to actively managing and reducing it. This therapeutic approach empowers individuals to take control of their health, fostering a sense of agency over their condition.

Implementing red light therapy requires consistency and patience. It's not a quick fix but rather a gradual process of healing and improvement. By committing to regular sessions and integrating complementary strategies like physical therapy and dietary adjustments, you can optimize your treatment outcomes. The key lies in persistence and adaptation—tailoring your approach based on how your body responds.

Incorporating red light therapy into your arthritis management plan offers a promising avenue for relief and enhanced mobility. Its ability to reduce inflammation and improve blood flow makes it an effective tool for easing joint pain and stiffness. Coupled with other strategies, it can significantly improve the quality of life for those living with arthritis. As you explore this therapeutic option, remember the value of a personalized approach tailored to your unique needs and circumstances.

MANAGING BACK PAIN: EFFECTIVE RED LIGHT STRATEGIES

Back pain, a common ailment affecting millions, often stems from muscle strain and spinal issues. Whether from heavy lifting, poor posture, or an existing condition, this discomfort can significantly impede daily activities. Muscle strain, characterized by overstretched or torn muscles, is a frequent culprit. It typically results from physical exertion or awkward movements, leaving the back vulnerable to pain. Red light therapy offers a promising solution by targeting these underlying causes with precision.

For effective back pain management, specific red light therapy protocols should be followed. Begin by positioning your device approximately six inches from the affected area to ensure optimal light penetration. Sessions should last between 15 and 20 minutes and be conducted three to five times a week. This frequency allows for cumulative benefits, promoting tissue repair and reducing inflammation. It's crucial to focus the therapy on areas of high tension or discomfort, such as the lower back or upper spine, depending on your specific needs. Consistency in application is key to achieving significant relief.

Incorporating ergonomic considerations alongside red light therapy enhances its effectiveness. Proper ergonomics, including maintaining good posture and using supportive equipment, play a critical role in preventing back pain recurrence. Adjust your work environment to support a neutral spine position, using chairs with adequate lumbar support and desks at comfortable heights. Invest in ergonomic accessories like footrests or standing desks to distribute weight evenly and reduce strain on your back. By integrating these practices with red light therapy, you create a holistic approach that addresses both symptom relief and prevention. Regular breaks to stretch and employ active sitting exercises can further alleviate ongoing stress on the spine, maintaining a balance between activity and rest.

Consider the case of John, a software engineer who suffered from chronic lower back pain due to long hours at his desk. After consulting with a specialist, he incorporated red light therapy into his routine. By following recommended protocols and making ergonomic adjustments at his workstation, John experienced significant improvements. He reported a reduction in pain levels and an increase in mobility after just a few weeks. His story highlights the power of combining therapy with lifestyle changes to achieve sustainable results.

Another illustrative example is Maria, a yoga instructor dealing with spinal alignment issues. Despite her active lifestyle, she faced persistent back pain that limited her practice. Through targeted red light therapy sessions focused on her lower spine and surrounding muscles, Maria found relief that allowed her to return to her full range of motion. Her experience underscores the versatility of red light therapy in managing various back pain causes and its ability to complement physical activity.

Integrative approaches can further enhance therapy effectiveness, such as combining red light therapy with massage therapy or acupuncture. These methods synergize well with the therapeutic red light, providing immediate relief and promoting long-term healing by continuing to improve blood circulation and muscle relaxation after sessions. Additionally, mindful movement practices like tai chi can offer gentle stretching and relaxation that complement red light therapy sessions, contributing to a comprehensive wellness approach.

The stories of individuals like John and Maria demonstrate the real-world impact of red light therapy on back pain management. They reveal how this non-invasive treatment can transform lives by providing relief from chronic discomfort. However, success requires dedication to consistent use and a willingness to adapt one's environment and habits for better ergonomic support.

To maximize the benefits of red light therapy for back pain, it's essential to remain proactive in your approach. Monitor your progress regularly, noting any changes in pain levels or mobility. Adjust your protocols as needed based on these observations, ensuring they remain aligned with your evolving needs. By taking an active role in managing your back pain, you empower yourself to alleviate symptoms and enhance your overall quality of life.

Red light therapy offers a promising pathway to effective back pain management through targeted protocols and ergonomic integration. Its ability to address common causes of discomfort positions it as a valuable tool for those seeking relief from the burdens of chronic back pain. By following recommended guidelines and learning from successful case studies, you can unlock its potential for healing and improved well-being.

REDUCING MUSCLE PAIN: TECHNIQUES FOR RELAXATION

Muscle pain often emerges from everyday activities or overexertion, a familiar foe for many. It typically stems from muscle tension and microtears, the latter being tiny injuries to the muscle fibers caused by overuse or sudden strain. These microtears, while small, can lead to significant discomfort as they heal, often resulting in stiffness and soreness. Red light therapy intervenes by accelerating the repair process of these microtears. It enhances cellular energy production, thereby boosting the efficiency of muscle recovery. This process eases existing pain and helps prevent future discomfort by improving overall muscle resilience.

For those seeking to alleviate muscle tension, specific protocols can enhance relaxation. Begin with a full-body session using red light therapy to promote overall relaxation. Position the device to cover large muscle groups like the back, thighs, and shoulders, maintaining a distance of about six to twelve inches. A session spanning 15 to 20 minutes, two to three times per week, can significantly reduce tension and promote relaxation. For more localized tension, focus on specific muscle groups. Target areas like the neck or lower back, adjusting the therapy duration to suit your needs. Regular application helps release tightness and encourages a sense of calm throughout the body.

Integrating red light therapy with other relaxation practices amplifies its benefits. Yoga, a practice grounded in mindfulness and physical awareness, complements red light therapy beautifully. Combining the two allows for a holistic approach to relaxation. Begin your session with gentle yoga stretches to warm up the muscles, followed by red light therapy to aid recovery and deepen relaxation. Deep breathing exercises further enhance this synergy. As you breathe deeply, your body enters a state of relaxation, optimizing the effects of the therapy. This combination not only alleviates muscle pain but also promotes mental clarity and emotional well-being.

The addition of visualization techniques can further amplify results, where imagining the light soothing sore muscles and revitalizing them adds a mental component to physical healing. Visualization helps in reducing stress levels, providing a dual benefit of calming the mind while easing physical discomfort.

Feedback from users illustrates the tangible benefits of these techniques. Consider Jane, an active retiree who experienced persistent muscle tension from gardening. She began using red light therapy alongside her yoga routine. After several weeks, she noticed a marked decrease in muscle soreness and an increase in her range of motion. Jane found that combining these practices relieved her physical discomfort and enhanced her overall quality of life. Similarly, Tom, a college athlete dealing with frequent muscle strain, incorporated red light therapy into his post-training routine. He reported reduced recovery time and less muscle stiffness, allowing him to maintain peak performance without extended downtime.

Testimonials like these highlight the real-world impact of integrating red light therapy with relaxation practices. They reveal how individuals across different lifestyles and age groups have found relief from muscle pain through consistent application and strategic combinations of therapy and exercise. The stories emphasize the importance of a tailored approach—one that considers personal habits and preferences to optimize results.

Through understanding muscle pain mechanisms and employing targeted protocols, you can effectively address tension and discomfort. Red light therapy serves as a powerful tool in your relaxation arsenal, offering relief from the strains of daily life. By integrating it with practices like yoga and deep breathing, you create a comprehensive plan for well-being that supports both physical and mental health. The journey towards reduced muscle pain is not only about finding immediate relief but also about fostering long-term wellness through thoughtful and intentional practices.

As someone who has explored various therapeutic methods throughout my career, I can attest to the profound impact that a comprehensive approach to pain management can have on one's life. Red light therapy offers a unique blend of science and simplicity, providing an accessible solution for those seeking to ease muscle pain and enhance relaxation. By focusing on the underlying causes of discomfort and employing targeted strategies, you empower yourself to live more comfortably and actively engage in the activities you love without being held back by muscle pain.

LONG-TERM PAIN MANAGEMENT PLANS: CONSISTENCY IS KEY

Imagine waking up one day, free from the persistent ache that shadows your every move. This vision can become reality with a consistent approach to red light therapy. Regular sessions form the backbone of effective long-term pain management. Establishing a routine is crucial; it's like setting a clockwork mechanism in motion. Consistency ensures that the therapeutic benefits accumulate over time, leading to sustained relief. Without a routine, you risk sporadic results that fail to address the root of your discomfort.

To build this routine, integrate red light therapy into daily life just as you would any other health practice. Choose a time that fits seamlessly into your schedule—perhaps early morning as part of your wake-up ritual or in the evening during relaxation. The key is regularity. Consistent exposure primes your body for healing, reinforcing the therapy's benefits each session. Over time, these small, consistent efforts yield substantial improvements in pain levels and overall well-being.

Tracking and monitoring your progress is equally important. A pain diary can serve as a valuable tool for this purpose. By documenting each session, noting the intensity of pain before and after, you create a record that helps identify patterns and triggers. This practice offers insights into what works best for you, allowing adjustments to your therapy protocols. Additionally, digital tools like apps can enhance this process. They provide reminders, track session frequency, and even offer visualization of progress over time. Such data-driven approaches empower you to make informed decisions about your therapy, tailoring it to suit your evolving needs.

Charting emotional states alongside physical symptoms can reveal connections between stress levels and pain experiences, further refining your therapy. This comprehensive approach ensures that you are addressing both mental and physical dimensions of chronic pain.

Adaptability remains a cornerstone of any successful long-term pain management plan. Pain doesn't remain static; it ebbs and flows with your life circumstances. Consequently, your therapy should also be flexible. Customize your plan based on the severity and frequency of your pain. On days when discomfort peaks, consider increasing session duration or intensity. Conversely, if you notice improvement, maintain regular sessions to sustain benefits without overexposure.

Success stories abound among those who have embraced this consistent approach. Take Linda, for instance. After years of struggling with fibromyalgia, she found solace in red light therapy. By adhering to a strict routine and diligently recording her progress, Linda managed to significantly reduce her pain levels. Her diary became a testament to her journey, capturing moments of triumph and setbacks alike. Over time, she learned to tweak her therapy sessions, finding the perfect balance that worked for her.

Similarly, Robert's experience with chronic migraines showcases the power of consistency. Initially skeptical, he began a disciplined regimen of red light therapy, meticulously tracking each session's impact on his headaches. Gradually, the frequency and intensity of his migraines diminished. This empowerment extended beyond physical relief; it restored his confidence in managing his condition independently.

These narratives highlight the transformative potential of consistent red light therapy. They demonstrate how individuals from diverse backgrounds have harnessed its benefits through dedication and adaptability. The common thread among them is not just the physical relief achieved but also the renewed sense of control over their lives. Moreover, they underscore the role of persistence and reflection in maximizing therapeutic outcomes.

As someone who has witnessed these transformations firsthand, I can attest to the power of consistency in pain management. Red light therapy offers a non-invasive, scientifically backed approach that empowers you to take charge of your health. By establishing a routine, tracking progress diligently, and adapting plans as needed, you pave the way for meaningful improvements in your quality of life.

Remember, success doesn't lie in the therapy itself but in how you integrate it into your daily life. Consistency serves as your ally—guiding each session towards long-term relief and enhanced well-being. Whether you're managing chronic conditions or seeking preventive care, a structured approach to red light therapy can unlock its full potential for healing and transformation.

Incorporating these practices into your routine requires commitment and patience. It's about making deliberate choices every day that prioritize your health and well-being. With time and perseverance, you too can experience the profound impact of consistent red light therapy on managing long-term pain effectively. This commitment to long-term health pays off in improved quality of life and greater daily functionality.

TESTIMONIALS: FINDING RELIEF WITH RED LIGHT THERAPY

In the realm of chronic pain management, personal stories illuminate the impact of red light therapy. Take, for instance, the account of Mary, a grandmother in her seventies, who had struggled with debilitating arthritis for over a decade. With regular red light therapy sessions, she experienced not only a decrease in joint pain but also a newfound ability to move with ease. Her pain level, once a constant eight on a ten-point scale, now rarely exceeds a three. This reduction has transformed her quality of life, allowing her to engage more actively with her grandchildren.

Similarly, consider the experience of Daniel, a high school athlete sidelined by persistent muscle pain. After incorporating red light therapy into his recovery routine, Daniel noted a marked improvement, both in terms of pain reduction and athletic performance. His quick recovery from injuries has bolstered his confidence, allowing him to return to his sport with renewed vigor. For Daniel, therapy provided not just physical relief but also emotional resilience, as his stress levels decreased and happiness increased.

These narratives are not isolated incidents; they reflect a broader trend of individuals across age groups finding solace in red light therapy. Quantifiable improvements include significant reductions in pain scales and enhanced mobility. Many users report that their pain levels dropped by several points on standard scales, shifting from severe discomfort to manageable levels. These changes are not just numbers but life-altering shifts that restore independence and vitality.

The emotional impacts of pain relief are profound. Chronic pain often casts a shadow over daily life, leading to frustration and diminished mental health. By alleviating this burden, red light therapy has facilitated increased happiness and reduced stress for many users. For people like Linda, a middle-aged office worker who struggled with back pain, the improvement in her physical state led to greater emotional well-being. She found herself more engaged at work and socially active, no longer held back by discomfort.

Visual documentation serves as compelling evidence of the therapy's effectiveness. Before-and-after photographs capture striking transformations in posture and expression, while pain management charts illustrate steady progress over time. Such documentation not only validates individual experiences but also provides encouragement to others considering this therapeutic option. Seeing tangible results motivates continued adherence to treatment protocols.

The role of community support cannot be understated in this context. Online forums and local support groups offer platforms for sharing experiences and advice, fostering a sense of solidarity among those navigating similar challenges. In these communities, individuals exchange insights on optimizing red light therapy and celebrate collective victories. This shared journey enhances motivation and accountability, reinforcing the positive impacts of therapy.

As we explore these stories, it becomes clear that red light therapy offers more than just symptomatic relief—it provides a pathway to rediscover life's pleasures without the constant hindrance of pain. The ripple effects extend beyond physical improvements, touching emotional and social dimensions. Users often find themselves reconnecting with activities they love and strengthening relationships once strained by their conditions.

In summary, testimonials from diverse individuals paint a vivid picture of red light therapy's potential to transform lives affected by chronic pain. Whether through quantifiable improvements or emotional liberation, the therapy offers hope and renewal across generations. As we conclude this chapter on managing chronic pain, let these stories inspire you to consider how red light therapy might integrate into your own life.

With this understanding in mind, we transition to our next topic—exploring how red light therapy can enhance cognitive function and mental clarity. This shift from physical to mental wellness highlights the therapy's versatility and underscores its role in holistic health management.

6

HOLISTIC HEALTH AND WELLNESS (EXPANDED EDITION)

ENHANCING SLEEP QUALITY: BETTER REST WITH RED LIGHT

Imagine the profound tranquility that envelops you during sleep, a state in which your mind, unfettered by stress, and your body, revitalized by rest, find harmony. While this dreamlike state remains elusive for many, red light therapy emerges as a beacon of science-backed promise, offering a novel approach to enhancing sleep quality. By understanding the fascinating complexities of sleep, we can appreciate how red light influences sleep cycles, promoting a deeper and more restorative slumber.

The heart of our sleep-wake patterns lies within the circadian rhythm, an internal clock governing our daily biological actions. Red light therapy plays a significant role in synchronizing this natural cycle by aligning exposure to ambient light, which directly affects the production of melatonin—an endocrine hormone pivotal in sleep regulation. Contrary to the disruptive blue light from electronics, red light creates a sleep-conducive environment by minimally interrupting melatonin production. This sets a biological stage for sleep readiness as bedtime draws near.

Detailed investigations into sleep patterns underscore the importance of natural light exposure in maintaining regular circadian cycles. Research highlights that red light, with its longer wavelengths, mimics the setting sun's hues, subtly signaling the brain that nighttime has arrived. Unlike artificial lighting often penetrating urban lives, red light remains harmonious with our evolutionary sleep cues, reinvigorating ancient sleep processes disrupted by modernity.

To effectively weave red light therapy into your bedtime rituals, it is essential to understand ideal timing and duration. Engaging in therapy sessions approximately 30 minutes before going to bed prepares your body to gracefully ease into relaxation. A session of about 10 to 20 minutes suffices to summon its beneficial effects without overstimulation. Placing your device at a comfortable range—such as beside your sleep space—facilitates effortless usage while ensuring optimal exposure. This considered approach can evolve into a cornerstone of your nightly routine, guiding you towards restorative relaxation.

Moreover, the quality of your sleep environment should not be underestimated. Creating a serene atmosphere by minimizing electronic usage and incorporating soothing scents can complement the calming nature of red light, rounding out an effective sleep routine. Aromatherapy with lavender or chamomile, for instance, may enhance the sense of calmness achieved through red light, inviting tranquility on multiple sensory levels.

For individuals afflicted with sleep disturbances such as insomnia or sleep apnea, red light therapy offers a potent complement to traditional management methods. By improving both sleep quality and duration, it can diminish symptoms related to these conditions. Although red light therapy is not a panacea, its integration with conventional treatments and lifestyle changes can yield significant improvements. For example, those with insomnia commonly struggle with initiating sleep; through consistent use, the gentle red hue can cue the brain towards rest, streamlining the transition into a nightly slumber.

Countless testimonials speak to the transformative power of red light therapy in altering sleep habits. Consider the case of Jane, a dynamic professional who grappled with stress-induced sleep interruptions. Her integration of red light therapy yielded not just improved sleep quality but also a reduction in wakeful periods during the night. Her narrative resonates with many who have adopted this therapy, highlighting its soothing influence as part of a comprehensive wellness strategy.

Interactive Element: Sleep Quality Tracking Journal

To fully leverage the red light therapy's sleep-enhancing potential, maintain a sleep quality journal to track progress. Document nightly routines, detailing the timing and duration of therapy sessions and the resultant changes in sleep patterns. Note specific elements such as ease of falling asleep and the frequency of night awakenings. Consistently keeping this journal provides valuable insights into your regimen's effectiveness, empowering you to make informed adjustments for ongoing improvement.

Incorporating feedback and observations from this journal into an iterative bedtime approach can amplify results. Experimenting with different light intensities, or varying the proximity and duration of sessions, may identify the optimal configuration for individual needs. Additionally, tracking dietary habits or stress levels alongside therapy results may uncover broader lifestyle factors influencing sleep, offering holistic insights into achieving restful nights.

Adopting red light therapy into your sleep rituals represents more than an addition; it's an investment in your comprehensive wellness. While exploring the benefits, remember that consistency is crucial. Take the opportunity to transition your nights from restless to rejuvenative, embracing this gentle and effective strategy for enhanced sleep quality.

BOOSTING MOOD AND ENERGY: LIGHTING UP YOUR DAY

Picture the morning sunlight, its gentle warmth signaling a fresh start to the day. Your daybreak can be further illuminated by red light therapy, providing an innovative approach to elevate mood and infuse energy. The scientific underpinning for this effect involves serotonin, a neurotransmitter fundamental to mood regulation. Red light exposure stimulates serotonin production, creating a ripple effect that uplifts well-being and energizes spirit. This lift offsets fatigue and inertia, morphing morning sluggishness into vitality and attentiveness.

Incorporating red light therapy in the morning hours can shape a positive, bustling day. To optimize its effects, blend the therapy with natural morning sunlight. Position your device wherever you savor your morning drink or breakfast, as a 10-minute session can invigorate you, mentally and physically priming you for the ensuing challenges. Embrace regular usage as a daily ritual for cumulative benefits, setting a positivity-filled and focused mind.

Refining the morning ritual to integrate mindfulness or meditative practices while exposed to red light can further augment its mood-lifting capabilities. A few minutes of meditation or positive affirmation techniques during light exposure help anchor tranquility, establishing a proactive mindset ready to tackle any endeavor.

For those afflicted with mood disorders, red light therapy extends supportive comfort. Seasonal Affective Disorder (SAD), triggered by reduced daylight exposure, entraps many in a cycle of melancholy and lethargy. Red light therapy mirrors natural sunlight's effects and alleviates SAD symptoms by recalibrating the internal clock and stabilizing mood changes. In addressing depression and anxiety, red light therapy, while not a standalone remedy, can complement other treatments, promoting mental well-being gently and non-invasively.

Personal accounts powerfully illustrate the influence of red light therapy on mood and vitality. Take, for example, Alex, who once waded through persistent energy dips and mood fluctuations during the shorter winter months. Following the introduction of red light therapy to his daily routine, Alex noted a significant uplift in his outlook and energy. He became more driven, less burdened by seasonal despair. Numerous individuals echo his success, finding optimism and vigor in red light's gentle illumination.

Similarly, the experiences of those who have integrated red light therapy with creative activities or exercise emphasize its wide-ranging potential. By pairing the therapy with morning yoga or a brisk walk, individuals report sustained energy levels and ameliorated creativity that persists throughout the day. This synthesis of physical activity with red light exposure demonstrates innovative approaches to harness augmented energy and mood.

INSPIRATIONAL STORY: A LIGHT IN THE DARK

Emily, an eager college student navigating academic pressures and social circles, unearthed red light therapy during her quest for natural energy enhancements. Initially skeptical, she incorporated it into her morning awakening habits. The shift was unmistakable; she became more alert, tackling classes with renewed vigor. Her previously variable mood stabilized, fortifying her emotional resilience and augmenting both personal interactions and academic successes. Emily's narrative underscores red light therapy's potential as a dependable ally for mental stability in life's daily challenges.

Translating Emily's experience to broader demographics, red light therapy holds promise beyond student life. Seniors pursuing active retirements, parents juggling household responsibilities, and professionals balancing demanding careers can all tailor red light integration to their routines. This adaptability makes the therapy universally appealing, capable of infusing daily life with vigor regardless of circumstances.

Exploring the integration of red light therapy into your life can enlighten paths to enhanced mood and vitality. By grasping its role in serotonin production to combat fatigue, informed choices facilitate its inclusion in wellness practices. Consistent use unveils a guiding light through dim days, aiding in navigation with enhanced ease and optimism.

Small shifts in daily habits can lead to noticeable life quality improvements. Embrace red light therapy as part of a comprehensive wellness approach, allowing it to highlight opportunities for revitalization and growth. Whether aiming for energy augmentation or mood support, red light therapy can provide the illumination needed to brighten every day with promise and potential.

SUPPORTING MENTAL CLARITY: FOCUS AND COGNITIVE BENEFITS

Red light therapy emerges as a promising avenue to enhance cognitive functioning, sharpen focus, and bolster memory. Central to its effects is neuroplasticity— the brain's remarkable ability to reorganize itself and form new neural connections. Such adaptability is crucial for learning, memory retention, and general mental agility. By amplifying neuroplasticity, red light therapy potentially heightens cognitive processes, facilitating the absorption of new information and its retrieval when necessary. Additionally, increased cerebral blood flow, augmented by red light exposure, supplies brain cells with essential oxygen and nutrients, backing optimal brain performance and improving everything from task execution to complex problem-solving.

For those seeking to enhance mental clarity through red light therapy, establishing a structured protocol is foundational. Typically, a regimen might involve sessions of 10 to 20 minutes, occurring multiple times weekly. Position the red light device at a comfortable distance, ensuring exposure across the forehead and temples. Sustained use is vital; the cumulative effects of regular installation yield discernible improvements in focus and memory. Scheduling these sessions during mental fatigue or before tackling cognitively intensive tasks can maximize benefits, providing a precise mental boost.

Ongoing research into the cognitive benefits of red light therapy yields encouraging outcomes. Studies showcase memory retention and mental acuity enhancements following regular red light exposure. One such study noted participants' improved ability to recall and understand new information after consistent therapy sessions (PMC). These findings highlight red light therapy's significant potential as a non-invasive means of supporting cognitive health, particularly for those experiencing age-related declines or cognitive burnout due to demanding lifestyles.

The tangible impact of red light therapy on cognition is best illustrated through personal experiences. Many report noticeable boosts in productivity and mental sharpness after incorporating regular red light sessions. Consider Mark—a middle-aged professional grappling with focus during long workdays. Post integration of red light into his morning routine, Mark found himself alert and efficient at work, with colleagues praising his heightened concentration and problem-solving. Such narratives illuminate the therapy's capacity to flip cognitive performance, offering hope to those seeking a natural mental clarity enhancement.

Integrating cognitive exercises or puzzles during red light exposure may further amplify cognitive benefits, engaging the mind actively while receiving optimized blood flow and nutrient delivery. Similarly, pairing red light with tasks that require sustained attention can lengthen focus endurance, making challenging projects more manageable and less taxing.

Visual Element: Cognitive Enhancement Infographic

Imagine an infographic delineating how red light therapy optimally supports cognitive function. The visual could showcase pathways by which cerebral blood flow increases and impacts neuroplasticity, furnishing a transparent representation of how red light boosts brain health. This tool would serve as an easy reference, reinforcing the necessity of consistency in seeking desired outcomes.

Beyond static resources, interactive cognitive mapping tools could illustrate individual progress over time. Logging personal achievements, cognitive milestones, or performing standardized tests within these tools could unveil nuanced insights into red light's long-term cognitive impact, providing motivation to maintain engagement.

Introducing red light therapy into cognitive wellness strategies provides an opportunity to natively enhance mental clarity. Whether as a student pursuing academic greatness, a professional chasing career elevation, or anyone desiring to maintain mental sharpness with age, this therapy offers a viable solution. By understanding its scientific basis and following systematic protocols, the full potential of red light therapy for cognitive development becomes accessible. Testimonials highlight its transformative powers and emphasize the potential achievable with dedication and consistent application of this groundbreaking mental wellness approach.

THE ROLE OF RED LIGHT IN STRESS REDUCTION

In modern existence, stress looms as a constant shadow, weaving into everyday life and fracturing peace. Red light therapy, a harbinger of balance, has emerged as a scientifically validated strategy to alleviate stress while nurturing relaxation. This therapy modulates cortisol—the hormone intricately associated with stress—as its central mechanism, helping to temper internal chaos and fostering a more harmonious inner ambiance. This modulation is crucial for individuals experiencing chronic stress, serving as a gentle yet potent means to temper the body's innate fight-or-flight response.

Furthermore, red light therapy activates the parasympathetic nervous system, colloquially known as the "rest and digest" system. This hits the brakes on stress-induced adrenaline surges, promoting recovery and positivity. As this system prevails, heart rates diminish, blood pressures level, and calmness abounds.

Embracing red light therapy into your regimen can create an oasis of tranquility amidst life's turmoil, steering your physiological state toward equilibrium.

To harness red light therapy effectively for stress mitigation, integrate it into guided meditations or breathing exercises. Begin by dedicating 15 to 20 minutes within a quiet environ where relaxation is uninterrupted. Set your red light device at a comfortable range to embrace its soothing rays. Inhale deeply, aligning your focus with the warmth and calming aura of the light. This ritual—practiced regularly—enhances the therapy's stress-mitigating potential and forges powerful harmonies with other calming practices.

Additionally, incorporating red light therapy into pre-sleep wind-down rituals can fortify stress resilience by soothing the mind before bedtime. Engaging the nervous system in a relaxation phase prior to rest can ensure a deep slumber, further supporting overall stress reduction. Pairing the therapy with reflective journaling or gratitude practices might deepen relaxation, promoting mental clarity and a positive outlook.

By merging red light therapy with additional stress-reduction practices, its benefits expand. Yoga and mindfulness complement red light's calming aura, anchoring you in the present and cultivating self-awareness. During yoga, incorporate brief red light exposure post-practice to accentuate relaxation and ease muscle recovery. Mindfulness users can use red light to anchor their meditation focus, enhancing serenity. These integrated approaches afford all-around stress management support, harmonizing mind and body movement.

As individuals share transformative stress-relief accounts via red light therapy, the therapy's impact becomes apparent. Imagine Sarah—a young professional feeling perpetually overwhelmed by work. Introducing red light therapy to her evening routine resulted in reduced anxiety and heightened tranquility. Sarah's narrative accentuates how this therapy can unwelcome life's stresses, aiding the restoration of inner balance and resilience.

David, a retiree wrestling with chronic health-related stress, found solace in red light therapy. A daily therapeutic practice offering respite from anxiety and instilling relaxation, the gentle red glow cherished, provided daytime tranquility upon daily conclusion. David's testimony underscores red light therapy's impressive capacity to promote well-being while alleviating contemporary life's stressors.

Interactive Element: Stress Relief Ritual Planner

Craft a personalized stress-relief ritual planner to integrate red light therapy meaningfully into everyday life. Outline dedicated therapy times and locations, combining them with relaxation preferences. Record emotional states pre- and post-session in conjunction with adjustments along the way. Over time, this planner becomes a vital tool to fine-tune methods and maximize the therapy's relaxation benefits.

Utilizing digital platforms to develop these planners might promote community interaction, inviting broader participation in red light therapy journeys. Sharing insights and strategies can generate a mutual-support network, cultivating collective growth and reinforcing the therapy's long-term viability.

Maximize red light therapy's stress-relief potential through consistent practice. Emphasizing regularity ensures cumulative advantages and solidifies commitment to self-care. As you explore aligning red light therapy with wellness initiatives, embrace experimentation and adaptation. Personalize practices based on unique needs and preferences, acknowledging individual variability.

Integrating this gentle yet profoundly impactful therapy invites tranquility and balance within life's demands and pressures. Understanding its mechanisms and pairing with complementary practices sets the stage for stress becoming serenity. Let red light therapy illuminate your journey toward a tranquil existence, a steadfast ally in the pursuit of holistic wellness.

7

ADVANCED INSIGHTS AND EMERGING RESEARCH

EXPLORING NEW WAVELENGTHS: BEYOND THE BASICS

The landscape of red light therapy, akin to a constantly shifting masterpiece, is evolving at a pace that can only be described as exhilarating. Like an artist experimenting with a new palette of colors to enhance creativity, the field of red light therapy is broadening its spectrum, pushing beyond the once-familiar territories of red and near-infrared wavelengths. This journey is comparable to setting sail into uncharted waters, lured by the promise of unveiling untapped potential and gaining a deeper understanding of the healing dimensions of light.

Researchers are delving into the realm of mid-infrared wavelengths, particularly in the 1000-1500 nm range, and are unearthing revolutionary paradigms. These wavelengths have been shown to penetrate deeper into the body than traditional wavelengths, suggesting groundbreaking possibilities, especially for patients with multifaceted medical conditions. Visualize light as a life-giving force, one that reaches into muscular layers and even permeates bones, facilitating distinct cellular processes that accelerate the recovery from chronic pain, significant injuries, and systemic ailments. Such advancements have the potential to redefine healthcare practices, bridging gaps where traditional methods encounter unyielding barriers, introducing a new frontier where light meets medicine in unprecedented ways.

On a molecular level, these emerging wavelengths interact in unique ways, presenting implications of great magnitude. Mid-infrared light, distinct from traditional wavelengths, is showing potential in modulating protein synthesis pathways, a crucial aspect of systemic repair and regeneration. Furthermore, it appears to influence the cellular communication systems that regulate inflammation and immune responses, positioning itself as a promising approach to myriad inflammatory conditions. Studies are emerging that suggest significant benefits for autoimmune diseases, where managing inflammation is pivotal for generating substantial improvements in health and quality of life.

Comparative analyses between traditional and mid-infrared wavelengths form a critical component of contemporary research. These studies dissect the distinct healing responses elicited by various wavelengths, offering critical insights into customized therapeutic methods. While traditional wavelengths are superior in epidermal treatments such as skin rejuvenation, their mid-infrared counterparts show potential in addressing issues that necessitate deeper intervention. The interplay between penetration depth and absorption highlights the importance of tailoring light therapy to specific therapeutic goals, such as targeting deep muscle recovery in athletes or facilitating tissue repair post-surgery. The potential for tailoring light treatment to an individual's unique physiological needs opens up a world of possibilities for personalized medicine, extending the benefits of red light therapy to previously unreachable strata of the health care spectrum.

Embarking on this quest to embrace new technological frontiers, though fraught with challenges, holds the promise of vast possibilities. The development of devices capable of delivering mid-infrared light safely and effectively demands breakthroughs in material science and is a challenging pursuit. This quest requires not just technical skill but also innovative thinking, compelling engineers to craft devices that are safe, user-friendly, and economically viable. Surmounting these challenges necessitates a continuous dialogue among researchers, pushing the boundaries of what is not only possible but also practical and sustainable, redefining our understanding of therapeutic modalities and applications permanently.

Interactive Element: Wavelength Exploration Exercise

Consider how expanding your knowledge of varied wavelengths can refine your treatment strategies. Maintain a comprehensive journal to track your health journey, setting ambitious goals and delineating the specific outcomes you aim to achieve with red light therapy. Routine reflections can deepen your comprehension of how various wavelengths might synchronize with your individual wellbeing aspirations, creating a personalized blueprint for ongoing health improvement.

As researchers push the boundaries of comprehension, the horizon of red light therapy remains expansive and enticing. By embracing new wavelengths and their biological interactions, we come ever closer to redefining the role of light in therapeutic practices. This relentless pursuit of knowledge encourages us to envision possibilities yet charted, fostering a spirit of curiosity and hope as we probe the mysteries of light and health, seeking innovative solutions to age-old challenges in health and wellness.

INNOVATIONS IN RED LIGHT TECHNOLOGY: WHAT'S NEXT?

Envision a future where red light therapy technology surpasses traditional limitations to establish groundbreaking paradigms in health and wellness. Recent technological advancements are reshaping this landscape, clearing pathways for more efficient and intuitive therapeutic solutions. The introduction of quantum dot technology marks a significant milestone. These nanometer-scale semiconductor particles offer precision and efficiency like never before, enabling meticulous customization of light wavelengths, dramatically transforming therapeutic outcomes and fostering personalized solutions perfectly aligned with specific health needs, whether for skin conditions, pain management, or holistic applications.

The integration of smart technology is set to revolutionize how users engage with red light therapy. Devices are evolving beyond mere instruments into adaptive, responsive systems that cater to individual user requirements. With app-controlled functionalities, users can effortlessly tune their therapy sessions to align with personal health initiatives. Imagine being empowered with real-time analytics on treatment efficiency, bolstered by data-driven insights that refine your approach over time. This synergy of intelligence and user control enhances therapy's effectiveness, embedding it seamlessly into modern life, giving users the ability to be at the helm of their health journeys and decisions.

Innovations in design and materials propel red light therapy devices toward unprecedented user-centered evolution. The advent of flexible, wearable designs exemplifies this trend, prioritizing ease of use and integration into daily routines. These devices are crafted from safe, lightweight materials, designed for prolonged contact without sacrificing comfort or efficacy. By merging resilience with user-centric designs, these innovations accommodate a broad spectrum of needs, whether users seek therapeutic interventions during extended activities or prefer quick, convenient sessions tailored to the demands of their busy lives.

A noteworthy industry shift is the burgeoning demand for home-use red light therapy devices, echoing a larger trend towards personalized health management, where individuals are taking proactive roles in overseeing their wellness. As the therapeutic benefits of red light therapy gain broader recognition, more consumers are incorporating it into their schedules from the comfort of their homes. The proliferation of accessible, high-quality devices democratizes this advanced therapy, making it more attainable to a wider audience and aligning with holistic health priorities, allowing people to take charge of their health and healing processes.

Reflecting on these technological strides reveals how they reimagine the future trajectory of red light therapy. Quantum dot enhancements elevate precision, while smart technology introduces unparalleled interactivity and customization. Advances in material science enhance comfort and convenience, fostering consistent usage and adherence. Market dynamics underscore a cultural shift towards home-based, accessible healthcare solutions that resonate with the philosophy of personalized wellbeing. As devices evolve, their ability to address a spectrum of health issues expands correspondingly, from superficial aesthetics to profound systemic interventions, enabling a comprehensive approach to personal health betterment.

The trajectory of red light therapy offers transformative potential across health spectrums, facilitated by continuous advancements. As you contemplate integrating these innovations into your health regimen, staying abreast of technological developments and industry trends is crucial. This awareness empowers you to fully harness red light therapy's benefits, allowing for informed choices that enhance your health journey. With each groundbreaking development, the promise of improved therapeutic outcomes strengthens, delivering nuanced and impactful solutions to both prevailing and nascent health challenges. As such, staying informed about the latest in red light therapy technology ensures you remain at the forefront of health innovations, poised to capitalize on its full spectrum of benefits tailored to your unique health requirements.

8

PRACTICAL IMPLEMENTATION AND LIFESTYLE INTEGRATION

BUILDING A ROUTINE: MAKING RED LIGHT PART OF YOUR DAY

Envision the gentle radiance of red light as an integral part of your daily rhythm, akin to the seamless flow of your morning ritual or nightly repose. Establishing a consistent routine is crucial for unlocking the myriad benefits of red light therapy. This regularity ensures a cumulative enhancement of your body's well-being, gradually reshaping your health landscape. Much like the benefits derived from daily physical activity or consuming a nutritionally balanced meal, regular red light therapy sessions forge a foundation for continuous wellness improvement.

Picture your daily schedule as a tapestry where moments of red light therapy embellish your life with self-care and vitality. In the invigorating dawn, utilize the revitalizing energy of red light to set a positive tone for your day. A concise 10-minute session can stimulate your senses, elevating both your mood and vitality. Integrate this practice while enjoying your morning brew, allowing the light to infuse you with invigoration. Alternatively, for those who prefer solace in the evening, red light therapy serves as a calming prelude to restful slumber. An evening session aligns with your body's circadian rhythm, enhancing relaxation and sleep quality (PMC, 2023).

To expand further on this idea, consider integrating red light therapy into meal preparation routines. While preparing dinner, let the soothing light envelop you, turning a routine task into a mindful retreat. The dual benefits of nourishing both your body with wholesome food and saturating yourself with therapeutic light create an environment of holistic wellbeing. This integration not only maximizes time but enriches daily activities with layers of wellness, fostering both physical health and mental clarity.

Incorporating these sessions into a bustling schedule might appear to be challenging, but strategic time management can simplify the process. Consider coupling therapy with existing activities such as meditation or reading. This concurrent approach maximizes your time, enabling unwinding alongside the therapeutic benefits of its gentle touch. Reflect on the day's happenings or indulge in a beloved novel while basking in the serene glow—creating a personal sanctuary at home.

Furthermore, introducing red light therapy during activities like your skincare regimen or post-workout cooldown can enhance its effectiveness. For instance, following a yoga session, when your muscles are unwinding, a short therapy duration can amplify relaxation, turning these moments into enriching breaks throughout your day.

For those who embrace creative outlets, red light therapy can be incorporated into your artistic pursuits. Imagine painting or sketching bathed in warm red light, where the serenity enhances focus and ignites creativity. This integration transforms artistic endeavors into a therapeutic experience, fostering a deeper connection with your craft and well-being.

Life's unpredictable nature often brings change, be it through travels or a shift in routines. Portable red light devices maintain your wellness consistency, wherever life takes you. These compact units fit effortlessly into your travel luggage, allowing therapy sessions to continue whether you're on a business trip or enjoying a family holiday. Staying adaptable during these times ensures that red light therapy remains your constant companion on your journey to optimal health.

Reflection Section: Designing Your Ideal Routine

Take a moment to reflect on how red light therapy can be seamlessly integrated into your everyday life. Craft a personalized schedule that aligns with your lifestyle and priorities. List possible time slots for therapy sessions and explore innovative ways to merge them with current activities. This reflection not only assists in planning but reiterates your dedication to enhancing well-being through deliberate integration.

Expand on this reflective practice by journaling these thoughts and creating a detailed map of your personal wellness journey. Visual organizers such as flowcharts or vision boards can be instrumental, transforming abstract thoughts into tangible plans, fostering accountability, and sustaining motivation.

As you embark on this path, let personalization be your guide. Recognize that what works for one person may differ for another, emphasizing the uniqueness of each routine in driving optimal results. By interweaving red light therapy into the daily fabric of your life, you pave the way for renewed physical and mental clarity.

Consider the use of visual aids, such as a dedicated section in a planner or calendar, to monitor your routine consistency. This method aids in maintaining regularity and provides a visual representation of your commitment and progress, serving as a motivational beacon.

Incorporating red light therapy into daily life is not merely about adding another task—it's about harmonizing technology with well-being. As you explore routines that resonate with you, remain open to adjustments that reflect changing needs and circumstances. This flexibility ensures that red light therapy becomes a steadfast pillar of health support in life's inevitable ebbs and flows.

OVERCOMING OBSTACLES: ADDRESSING COMMON CHALLENGES

Embarking on red light therapy can initially involve challenges that seem daunting. Time constraints are often formidable. In our modern fast-paced world, dedicating moments to self-care can feel overwhelming amidst a deluge of responsibilities. The day's demands—from professional commitments to familial obligations—often leave scant room for additional practices. Motivation may also wane when results aren't immediately visible. It's easy to feel thwarted when change is gradual, impacting consistency.

To circumvent these hurdles, consider practical strategies like creating a designated self-care corner in your home where therapy can seamlessly fit amid daily life routines. This designated area, perhaps accentuated with calming decor, can become a go-to space, reinforcing the habit's importance and ease of access.

Nurture a mindset of patience and perseverance; therapy's gradual nature does not diminish its cumulative benefits. Understand the value of minor shifts and acknowledge them as progress. Consider documenting these subtle changes in a journal to remind yourself that progress, albeit slow, is being made.

Mindset is pivotal in successfully incorporating red light therapy into your life. Cultivating a positive outlook can transform this practice from an obligation into an opportunity for growth. Setting realistic expectations is crucial. Recognize that immediate transformations may not be apparent, but their gradual build-up over time will be significant. Goals should be attainable, emphasizing progressive improvement over instant perfection. This approach reduces frustration, enhances motivation, and keeps you aligned with your wellness objectives.

Exploring the concept of mindfulness can further solidify this outlook. Engaging in brief mindfulness meditations before or after sessions can fortify the therapy's psychological benefits. These moments encourage reflection on personal growth, fostering gratitude and awareness.

Connect with others navigating similar obstacles, offering a rich tapestry of shared experiences and solutions. Mark, for example, is a busy professional who initially found time management difficult. By setting small, achievable goals and maintaining a positive mindset, he successfully incorporated red light therapy into his routine, leading to improved energy levels and skin health. Similarly, Sarah experienced motivational slumps but discovered that creating a peaceful therapy space revitalized her commitment. These narratives highlight the resilience necessary to overcome initial barriers, reminding us of the rewarding outcomes that persistence often yields.

Engagement with supportive networks extends beyond motivational reinforcement; it allows for sharing strategies and solutions, offering new perspectives from those who have overcome similar obstacles.

MOTIVATIONAL TESTIMONIAL: A CASE OF RESILIENCE

Consider Emma's journey, a testament to adaptability and resilience. Initially skeptical about the time commitment required, she found herself overwhelmed by competing priorities. Yet, she embraced the challenge, setting reminders on her phone to signal therapy sessions amidst her hectic schedule. Gradually, she transformed her living room into a calming oasis for red light therapy—a place accentuated with gentle lighting and comfortable seating. This environmental shift rekindled her motivation, turning each session into a cherished ritual rather than an obligation.

Emma's ongoing adaptation included integrating her passion for reading with therapy, setting aside a particular book only for her sessions. This pairing of enjoyment with care reinforced her dedication and became a delightful aspect she anticipated daily.

Emma's story underscores the importance of mindset and environment in achieving success. Her initial skepticism morphed into enthusiasm as she observed meaningful albeit subtle changes in her well-being. Not only did her skin become more radiant, but she also experienced improved clarity and focus during her workday. Emma's transformation illustrates that overcoming obstacles requires practical adjustments alongside an unwavering commitment to personal growth.

In tackling common challenges, it is essential to remember that each individual's journey is unique. Flexibility in approach and adaptability of mindset are key to successfully integrating red light therapy into life. By acknowledging obstacles and embracing solutions, you lay the foundation for lasting transformation. Whether through technical aids like reminders or creating a nurturing home environment, these strategies empower you to navigate challenges with confidence and grace.

Ultimately, the path to integrating red light therapy is not without its trials. Yet, it is through these challenges that we discover our potential for resilience and growth. As you embark on this endeavor, remain mindful of the inner power you possess to overcome obstacles and cultivate a lifestyle celebrating health and vitality. With each session, you inch closer to your wellness aspirations—fortified by determination and inspired by the successes of others who have walked this illustrious path before you.

MONITORING PROGRESS: TRACKING RESULTS FOR MOTIVATION

Incorporating red light therapy into your daily life is a journey of discovery and transformation, where tracking progress significantly enhances both motivation and effectiveness. Observing how your body responds to therapy can offer invaluable insights, rendering your progress into a visible map of improvement. It becomes a narrative where even the most minute changes are celebrated milestones. By documenting these alterations, you foster a sense of achievement and clarity, serving as a powerful motivator to persist in your efforts.

Consider developing a tailored progress chart, inclusive of baseline health measurements and specific goals like energy levels or skin tone. Such charts visually delineate growth, providing tangible proof of therapy's impact over time.

Visual tracking of improvements provides a tangible record of your journey, reinforcing progress and enthusiasm. Observing changes over time strengthens the perceived impact of the therapy, aiding in maintaining enthusiasm and commitment. Reduction in pain levels or visible skin improvements are essential indicators of success. They validate your efforts and guide therapy optimizations. Such tracking offers a baseline against which progress is measured, helping you refine your approach for maximum benefit.

Leveraging technological tools to track your progress can provide a comprehensive overview, reinforcing motivation. Consider utilizing health and wellness apps that allow easy data entry and goal setting, which can be synced with other health metrics to give a holistic view of improvements.

To effectively track progress, consider leveraging apps and digital journals designed for wellness monitoring. These tools allow you to log sessions, note changes, and compare results over time. Digital platforms often include features like reminders and trend analysis, guiding your course. Additionally, maintaining a therapy log detailing session duration, frequency, and personal observations can be immensely beneficial. This log becomes a living document that chronicles your journey, capturing nuances that might otherwise go unnoticed.

Incorporating health metrics beyond physical changes, like stress reduction or sleep quality, further deepens understanding of therapy's comprehensive benefits. This broad perspective enriches personal insights and adjustments.

Focus on key metrics like pain level reduction and skin appearance changes. Documenting pain fluctuations can unveil patterns related to therapy sessions, offering crucial insights into what works best for you. Similarly, tracking skin changes—be it enhanced elasticity or reduced blemishes—provides concrete evidence of progress. These observations equip you to make informed decisions about session adjustments, ensuring therapy aligns with evolving needs.

By leveraging feedback tools, both internal reflections and external apps offer a robust tracking mechanism, refining each session's effectiveness by celebrating triumphs and identifying recalibration areas.

Regular reviews of tracked data are vital for maintaining momentum and effectiveness. Monthly assessments allow you to evaluate progress comprehensively, offering insights into successful strategies or areas needing adjustment. Such periodic reflection helps prevent stagnation, keeping therapy dynamic and responsive to your body's needs. By reviewing data consistently, you foster an environment of continuous improvement, with each session building on the last.

Interactive Element: Progress Tracking Exercise

Consider engaging in a progress tracking exercise to deepen your understanding of therapy's impact. Begin by selecting specific metrics to monitor—such as pain levels, skin appearance, or energy changes—and record them consistently over a month. At this period's end, review your entries to identify patterns and insights. This exercise enhances motivation and equips you with knowledge to adapt therapy for optimal results.

Expand this exercise by sharing your results in a community forum, where comparisons and discussions with other users can enhance understanding and stimulate new strategies for effectiveness.

Encourage collaboration with peers during this exercise by sharing findings and insights. This collective knowledge exchange not only broadens understanding but solidifies connections within the red light therapy community.

Tracking progress transforms red light therapy from passive activity to active wellness pursuit. By engaging with your data, you take ownership of your health journey, making informed decisions reflecting your unique needs and goals. This proactive approach fosters a deeper connection with therapy, reinforcing its role as an integral lifestyle component.

Embracing tracking as a motivational tool illuminates the path ahead and honors the strides made along the way. It shifts focus from destination to discovery, where each recorded change celebrates your commitment and perseverance. This practice reaffirms therapy's value and potential, inspiring continued engagement with a renewed purpose.

Incorporate reflective journaling to accompany data tracking, providing qualitative depth to quantitative metrics and enriching the holistic wellness narrative.

As you embark on monitoring progress, remember that every log entry tells a story—your transformation through red light therapy. The act of tracking becomes an empowering ritual grounding you in the present while guiding future actions. With each entry, you forge a deeper connection with your well-being, nurturing an environment where growth and exploration naturally flourish.

Though no two experiences are exactly alike, the common thread woven through each account is resilience and determination. Like red light penetrating deeply to promote healing, so too does monitoring penetrate the surface, revealing underlying truths about our health journey. Every recorded observation brings greater clarity—a clarity illuminating possibilities for continuous growth and improvement through red light therapy's enduring promise.

ENCOURAGING EXPERIMENTATION: PERSONALIZING YOUR APPROACH

Experimentation with red light therapy opens a gateway to discover the best approach for yourself. Every person's needs and responses are distinct, and experimentation allows you to customize therapy to your individual requirements. Trying out different session lengths and frequencies can reveal the perfect balance for your body. Some might find shorter, more frequent sessions invigorating, while others benefit from longer, less frequent exposure. Such personalization is crucial as it aligns therapy with your unique rhythms and health objectives.

Expand your experimentation framework by introducing diverse settings and curating an environment conducive to trial and error, which aids in refining therapy protocols that resonate with your personal health aspirations.

When adjusting therapy, prioritize safety. Begin with gradual modifications in intensity and duration to gauge your body's response. Start with recommended settings and incrementally increase them, observing any changes in comfort or effectiveness. This cautious approach minimizes the risk of overexposure while maximizing benefits. Listen to your body's signals as they guide you towards the most advantageous protocol. You may detect subtle shifts post-session, informing future adjustments.

Integrate feedback loops within experiments, documenting body responses to different settings, fostering a nuanced understanding of what suits your wellness journey best.

Beyond standard sessions, contemplate integrating red light therapy creatively into various daily life aspects. Perhaps your morning yoga routine could be elevated by incorporating red light therapy, enhancing meditative effects. Envision yourself immersed in a gentle glow while practicing yoga poses, deepening relaxation and focus. Alternatively, consider therapy during a soothing evening bath, creating a tranquil sanctuary rejuvenating both mind and body.

Expand these creative integrations into unexpected daily activities, uncovering spaces where therapy can seamlessly intertwine with life's tasks, amplifying wellness benefits.

Creativity can extend beyond conventional wellness practices. Envisage using red light therapy during mundane tasks like folding laundry or writing emails. These moments become opportunities for self-care, transforming routine activities into therapeutic experiences. By embracing such innovative applications, you frame everyday life into a canvas for wellness exploration, enriching your relationship with red light therapy.

Success stories abound from those embracing experimentation, illustrating the power of personalized approaches. Lisa, who initially battled persistent muscle tension, found relief by merging therapy with her nightly stretching routine. The synergy between light exposure and physical movement amplified results, easing tension more effectively than either method alone.

Similarly, Tom succeeded by experimenting with session timing. Although evening sessions offered limited benefits initially, switching to mornings revolutionized his experience, energizing him for the day. This shift underscores the importance of adaptability in finding what suits individual lifestyles and needs best.

Embrace multifaceted approaches that amalgamate therapy with distinct practices, such as breath work or cognitive exercises, expanding wellness dimensions while enhancing therapy effectiveness.

Another compelling narrative comes from Emily, who integrated therapy into her creative pursuits as an artist. Using red light during painting sessions, the ambient glow became part of her creative process, enhancing focus and productivity. Emily's experience exemplifies how red light therapy transcends conventional boundaries, becoming an integral component of diverse activities.

These narratives demonstrate that personalization fosters deeper connections with red light therapy, uncovering possibilities beyond standard protocols. They emphasize the importance of curiosity and openness in maximizing the therapy's potential. By embracing experimentation, you embark on a path of self-discovery, where each session holds potential for new insights and enhanced well-being.

Encourage yourself to explore the uncharted territory of personalized red light therapy. Challenge assumptions about what constitutes a typical session, redefining it to reflect your lifestyle and preferences. This process transforms therapy from a static routine into a dynamic interaction evolving with you. Through experimentation, you unlock a spectrum of possibilities that enhancement extends beyond physical health to include creativity and enjoyment in daily life.

Consider establishing a documentation habit during experimentation phases, enriching future adjustments with a comprehensive history of tested variables and their outcomes.

In crafting your personalized approach to red light therapy, remember flexibility is key. Allow room for adaptation as you learn more about your body's responses and preferences. Each session becomes an opportunity for exploration—a chance to refine and redefine what wellness signifies for you. Embrace this freedom to experiment and discover, knowing this process holds potential for profound transformation and growth.

COMMUNITY AND SUPPORT: CONNECTING WITH FELLOW USERS

Engaging with a community of fellow red light therapy users can immensely enrich your experience. These connections offer a tapestry of shared experiences and wisdom that are both comforting and enlightening. Joining such a community transcends mere mutual interest; it becomes a space where collective knowledge thrives. Here, you can exchange tips, share successes, and learn from others' challenges. This learning environment fosters growth and motivation, refining your therapy approach for greater effectiveness and alignment with your needs.

Maximize engagement by exploring diverse community platforms, including online and local forums, to locate a group resonating with your therapeutic vision and goals.

There are numerous venues for connecting with other red light therapy followers. Online forums and social media groups serve as popular platforms where users gather to discuss their journeys. These digital spaces are accessible and convenient, enabling you to engage with others regardless of location. They provide opportunities to ask questions, share experiences, and receive feedback from a diverse group. Additionally, you may find local wellness meetups or workshops focusing on holistic health practices, including red light therapy. These gatherings offer face-to-face interactions, encouraging deeper connections and personalized advice.

Strategize dynamic interaction opportunities by engaging community leaders or experienced members, leveraging their insights for therapy enhancement and personal growth.

The benefits of being part of such a community extend beyond mere information exchange. Learning from others' experiences can invigorate your therapy routine, introducing techniques or approaches you haven't considered. Observing others overcome a plateau or integrate therapy into unconventional routines can inspire creativity in your practice. Success stories within these communities act as motivators, emphasizing what's achievable through persistence and dedication. As you learn from peers, your understanding and application of red light therapy evolve.

Implement a strategy for reciprocal learning within community exchanges by offering your insights and experiences while benefiting from others' wisdom, enhancing communal growth.

Consider Paul's story, who initially struggled with therapy consistency. Feeling isolated, he joined an online red light therapy group. The community's support transformed his approach; members shared tips that helped establish a lifestyle-compatible routine. More importantly, Paul found accountability partners who motivated him to keep on track. Their encouragement led to noticeable improvements in his energy and skin health, reinforcing community engagement's value.

Communities also provide accountability. When you share your goals, you create a network invested in your progress, fostering responsibility—not just to yourself but also to supporters. This shared commitment enhances perseverance through challenges, transforming solitary efforts into collaborative endeavors, where collective success is celebrated.

For others, a community's impact transcends motivation, becoming a lifeline nurturing resilience and perseverance. Take Sarah, for example. Facing skepticism from family dampened her enthusiasm for therapy effectiveness. Seeking validation, she connected with a local wellness group that welcomed her. The group's belief in holistic health empowered her to continue with renewed vigor. Their success stories bolstered her confidence, helping her achieve once unattainable results.

Maintain consistent community interaction, contributing feedback and experiences to fortify connections, thus weaving a robust network of shared success stories.

Connecting with fellow users enhances emotional well-being. The belonging stemming from shared interests forms bonds transcending geographic boundaries. Through these connections, you gain not only advice but friendship and support, enriching your red light therapy journey by transforming it into a communal health celebration.

Active participation in such communities can be as simple as sharing weekly progress or offering encouragement to others facing similar challenges. These reciprocal interactions strengthen community bonds while enriching your journey. Whether through digital platforms or local meetups, the connections you forge become integral to your therapeutic practice.

For more in-depth community engagement, organize informal virtual meetups or discussions, reflecting on shared challenges and celebrating collective successes, enhancing relational intimacy.

Embracing this community aspect of red light therapy opens you to a world of shared knowledge and support. It becomes an opportunity to learn not just about therapy but about perseverance, resilience, and the collective growth power. Through engagement, you find wellness allies—individuals who inspire and uplift as you navigate the health path together.

SUSTAINING LONG-TERM BENEFITS: COMMITMENT TO WELLNESS

In the realm of red light therapy, lasting benefits rest on a foundation of steadfast commitment. While this therapy offers remarkable potential, its full spectrum of advantages unfolds gradually. Sustained dedication is the key, where each session builds upon previous ones, weaving a tapestry of improved health and vitality. The process mirrors nurturing a garden, where patience and consistency yield flourishing results. Recognizing that changes may initially be subtle is crucial. Like a bud's slow unfolding, red light therapy's benefits manifest over time, requiring perseverance and faith in the process.

Integrate long-term strategy adjustments based on periodic evaluations, aligning commitment with evolving life circumstances, ensuring sustainability and efficacy.

Maintaining long-term engagement involves setting and revisiting wellness goals. These goals act as guiding stars, illuminating your sustained improvement path. As objectives are defined, consider how red light therapy can support them. Are you seeking enhanced energy, clearer skin, or reduced pain? Regularly revisiting these goals helps remain focused and motivated, allowing for adjustments as needs evolve. Celebrating milestones underscores your commitment, providing tangible progress proof. Whether it's decreased joint discomfort or a mood boost, acknowledging these achievements fuels continuation motivation.

Regular goal assessment ensures therapy aligns with life's shifting dynamics, fostering adaptability crucial for maintaining long-term engagement.

Integrating red light therapy into a broader wellness strategy enhances effectiveness, creating a holistic health approach addressing various well-being facets. Pairing therapy with balanced nutrition ensures essential nutrients for cellular repair and rejuvenation. A diet rich in antioxidants and vitamins complements the therapy's antioxidative effects, enhancing overall benefits. Regular physical activity amplifies results by promoting circulation and muscle health. Simple exercises like walking or stretching align with therapy, fostering a comprehensive wellness approach that nurtures both body and mind.

Deepen wellness integration by exploring symbiotic practices, harmonizing therapy with unconventional health modalities like acupuncture or naturopathy for holistic balance.

Mental health practices play an equally vital role in this equation. Techniques such as mindfulness and meditation create a serene mental space complementing physical treatments. They manage stress and enhance mental clarity, reinforcing red light therapy's positive impact. Together, these elements form a robust wellness plan sustaining long-term benefits. By embracing this integrated approach, a lifestyle supporting continuous improvement is created, where each component strengthens the others.

Long-term success stories showcase red light therapy's transformative power through commitment. Consider Nancy, who embarked on this path to alleviate chronic pain—her journey emblematic of resilience and dedication. Over months, she experienced significant pain reduction and improved mobility. Nancy's unyielding commitment transformed her physical health while revitalizing her spirit, allowing fuller engagement with life's activities. Similarly, David's experience underscores the cumulative effects of sustained therapy. Initially seeking brighter skin, he discovered enhanced energy and mood as unexpected benefits. David's journey illustrates how dedication unlocks unforeseen advantages enriching daily life.

As practitioners of long-term wellness explore these integration stories, establishing a framework for evaluating their own goals and aspirations could enhance therapy's transformative potential.

These testimonials illuminate perseverance's profound impact in achieving wellness goals through red light therapy. They remind us that while the path requires patience, the rewards are substantial. Each story reinforces that sustained effort yields lasting transformation, inspiring others to remain steadfast in their health pursuit.

As this chapter concludes, remember that commitment is the cornerstone of realizing red light therapy's potential. It requires a holistic perspective embracing both physical and mental well-being, fostering a health-thriving environment. The journey towards sustained benefits involves intention and action, rooted in understanding wellness as a dynamic process necessitating continuous investment.

Share insights from your journey with nascent users, offering guidance and encouragement, forming legacy narratives empowering continual growth across the therapy community.

Looking ahead to our next chapter, we will explore how technological advancements continue shaping and expanding red light therapy possibilities. As we delve into this remarkable tool's future, contemplate how today's commitment lays tomorrow's innovations and discoveries foundation—enhancing health and vitality.

CONCLUSION

As we reach the culmination of this enlightening journey through red light therapy, I invite you to pause and reflect on the rich tapestry of knowledge we have woven together. From the ancient sunlit healing rituals of Egypt to the cutting-edge scientific breakthroughs of today, you have explored the profound potential of red light therapy. This book has served as a comprehensive guide, delving into its myriad applications—from skin rejuvenation to enhancing physical performance, and from pain management to holistic wellness.

Throughout this exploration, we have uncovered the science underpinning red light therapy. You've learned about its ability to stimulate cellular repair, reduce inflammation, and promote overall health. The historical evolution and scientific mechanisms of red light therapy have been laid bare, offering a solid foundation upon which to build your understanding. Key strategies and practical applications have been detailed, equipping you with tools to harness its benefits for your own well-being.

The insights gained from this book are not merely theoretical but are designed to be actionable. Whether you're addressing specific health concerns or seeking to enhance your overall vitality, the strategies outlined here are intended for real-world application. The importance of selecting the right equipment, understanding the science behind wavelengths, and tailoring protocols to your unique needs are all critical components of this journey. Remember, the key takeaways are your guideposts as you venture into the world of red light therapy.

My motivation for writing this book was deeply personal. As a retired Sports Chiropractor, I've spent decades searching for and applying effective natural therapies. My experiences have shown me the transformative power of non-invasive, science-backed treatments. Red light therapy stands out as a particularly potent tool, and my desire is to empower you with this knowledge. My hope is that you will feel equipped and inspired to integrate these practices into your life, leading to enhanced wellness and vitality.

The journey doesn't end here. I encourage you to continue exploring red light therapy beyond these pages. The field is ever-evolving, with new research and innovations emerging regularly. Stay curious, remain open to experimentation, and tailor your approach as you discover what works best for you. Your proactive engagement with red light therapy will benefit your health and contribute to the broader understanding of its potential.

As you embark on this next phase of your wellness journey, consider the impact of sharing your experiences with others. Your insights and results could inspire friends, family, or community members to explore red light therapy for themselves. Through these shared experiences, you can contribute to a growing movement towards natural, effective healthcare solutions.

In closing, let me leave you with an inspirational message: the power to transform your health is within your reach. Red light therapy is a remarkable tool that, when used thoughtfully, can enhance your life in meaningful ways. Embrace the knowledge and tools you've acquired, and use them to create a wellness routine that supports your goals. May your journey be filled with renewed energy, vibrant health, and the joy of discovering what is possible when you align modern science with the wisdom of natural healing.

Thank you for joining me on this exploration. Here's to a future where light illuminates our surroundings and enriches our lives.

REFERENCES

Niels Ryberg Finsen – Facts https://www.nobelprize.org/prizes/medicine/1903/finsen/facts/

Photobiomodulation—Underlying Mechanism and Clinical ... https://pmc.ncbi.nlm.nih.gov/articles/PMC7356229/

Photobiomodulation CME part I: Overview and mechanism ... https://www.sciencedirect.com/science/article/abs/pii/S0190962224001865

Red Light Therapy: Uses, Benefits, and Risks https://www.healthline.com/health/red-light-therapy

We Wanted to Find the Best Red Light Therapy Device ... https://www.nytimes.com/wirecutter/reviews/red-light-therapy-devices/

Red Light Wavelength: Everything You Need to Know https://platinumtherapylights.com/blogs/news/red-light-wavelength-everything-you-need-to-know?

We Wanted to Find the Best Red Light Therapy Device ... https://www.nytimes.com/wirecutter/reviews/red-light-therapy-devices/

8 Best Red-Light Therapy Devices 2025, Tested ... - Glamour https://www.glamour.com/gallery/best-red-light-therapy-devices

Reverse skin aging signs by red light photobiomodulation https://pmc.ncbi.nlm.nih.gov/articles/PMC10311288/

9 ways to stimulate collagen production in skin https://www.medicalnewstoday.com/articles/317151

Red light phototherapy alone is effective for acne vulgaris https://pubmed.ncbi.nlm.nih.gov/17903156/

Red Light Therapy For Dark Spots | Blog https://www.solawave.co/blogs/red-light-therapy/red-light-therapy-for-dark-spots

Photobiomodulation in human muscle tissue https://pmc.ncbi.nlm.nih.gov/articles/PMC5167494/

Photobiomodulation in human muscle tissue https://pmc.ncbi.nlm.nih.gov/articles/PMC5167494/

Red Light Therapy: What it is and Uses for Athletes by Liam ... https://www.athleticlab.com/red-light-therapy-for-athletes/

CrossFit Athletes Share Their Experience With Red Light ... https://kineon.io/blogs/news/red-light-therapy-crossfit?

Low-intensity LASER and LED (photobiomodulation ... https://pmc.ncbi.nlm.nih.gov/articles/PMC9980499/

Can osteoarthritis be treated with light? https://arthritis-research.biomedcentral.com/articles/10.1186/ar4354

Infrared therapy for chronic low back pain: A randomized ... https://pmc.ncbi.nlm.nih.gov/articles/PMC2539004/

Red Light Therapy: Effectiveness, Treatment, and Risks https://www.webmd.com/skin-problems-and-treatments/red-light-therapy

Effects of red light on sleep and mood in healthy subjects ... https://pmc.ncbi.nlm.nih.gov/articles/PMC10484593/

Red Light Therapy for Depression https://timewellnesscenters.com/red-light-therapy-for-depression/

Significant Improvements in Cognitive Performance Post ... https://pmc.ncbi.nlm.nih.gov/articles/PMC4043367/

Red-Light Therapy for Stress Relief: A Natural Solution at ... https://www.redlighttherapycenter.com/blog/red-light-therapy-for-stress-relief

A Controlled Trial to Determine the Efficacy of Red and ... https://pmc.ncbi.nlm.nih.gov/articles/PMC3926176/

Quantum dot light-emitting diodes as light sources in ... https://iopscience.iop.org/article/10.1088/2515-7639/ab95e8

Photobiomodulation (PBM) Devices - Premarket ... https://www.fda.gov/regulatory-information/search-fda-guidance-documents/photobiomodulation-pbm-devices-premarket-notification-510k-submissions

Photobiomodulation Research | The Barron Lab https://barronlab.stanford.edu/research/photobiomodulation-research

How to Incorporate Red Light Therapy into Your Daily Routine https://havenofheat.com/blogs/red-light-therapy-guides/incorporate-red-light-therapy-daily-routine

7 Time Management Skills To Improve Your Mental Health https://psychcentral.com/health/tips-to-improve-your-time-management-skills

Maximizing the Benefits of Red-Light Therapy https://www.redlighttherapycenter.com/blog/maximizing-the-benefits-of-red-light-therapy-the-power-of-tracking-your-progress

Made in the USA
Monee, IL
04 November 2026

67385800R00075